States of Mind
Configurational Analysis
of Individual Psychology

SECOND EDITION

CRITICAL ISSUES IN PSYCHIATRY
An Educational Series for Residents and Clinicians

Series Editor: Stephen Scheiber, M.D.
Northwestern University
Evanston, Illinois

Recent volumes in the series:

CLINICAL DISORDERS OF MEMORY
Aman U. Khan, M.D.

CLINICAL PERSPECTIVES ON THE SUPERVISION OF
PSYCHOANALYSIS AND PSYCHOTHERAPY
Edited by Leopold Caligor, Ph.D., Philip M. Bromberg, Ph.D.,
and James D. Meltzer, Ph.D.

CONTEMPORARY PERSPECTIVES ON PSYCHOTHERAPY WITH
LESBIANS AND GAY MEN
Edited by Terry S. Stein, M.D., and Carol J. Cohen, M.D.

DIAGNOSTIC AND LABORATORY TESTING IN PSYCHIATRY
Edited by Mark S. Gold, M.D., and A. L. C. Pottash, M.D.

DRUG AND ALCOHOL ABUSE: A Clinical Guide to Diagnosis
and Treatment, Second Edition
Marc A. Schuckit, M.D.

EMERGENCY PSYCHIATRY: Concepts, Methods, and Practices
Edited by Ellen L. Bassuk, M.D., and Ann W. Birk, Ph.D.

ETHNIC PSYCHIATRY
Edited by Charles B. Wilkinson, M.D.

MOOD DISORDERS: Toward a New Psychobiology
Peter C. Whybrow, M.D., Hagop S. Akiskal, M.D., and
William T. McKinney, Jr., M.D.

NEUROPSYCHIATRIC FEATURES OF MEDICAL DISORDERS
James W. Jefferson, M.D., and John R. Marshall, M.D.

THE RACE AGAINST TIME: Psychotherapy and Psychoanalysis
in the Second Half of Life
Edited by Robert A. Nemiroff, M.D., and Calvin A. Colarusso, M.D.

STATES OF MIND: Configurational Analysis of Individual
Psychology, Second Edition
Mardi J. Horowitz, M.D.

TREATMENT INTERVENTIONS IN HUMAN SEXUALITY
Edited by Carol C. Nadelson, M.D., and David B. Marcotte, M.D.

A Continuation Order Plan is available for this series. A continuation order will bring
delivery of each new volume immediately upon publication. Volumes are billed only
upon actual shipment. For further information please contact the publisher.

States of Mind

Configurational Analysis
of Individual Psychology

SECOND EDITION

Mardi J. Horowitz, M.D.

University of California at San Francisco
San Francisco, California

Plenum Medical Book Company • New York and London

Library of Congress Cataloging in Publication Data

Horowitz, Mardi Jon, 1934–
    States of mind.

    (Critical issues in psychiatry)
    Bibliography: p.
    Includes index.
    1. Psychotherapy. 2. Psychoanalysis. 3. Personality. I. Title. II. Title: Configurational
analysis of individual psychology. III. Series. [DNLM: 1. Psychoanalysis. 2. Psychotherapy.
WM 460 H8165s]
RC480.H64   1987   616.89′14   87-2571
ISBN 0-306-42449-5

© 1987 Mardi J. Horowitz, M.D.

Plenum Medical Book Company is an imprint
of Plenum Publishing Corporation
233 Spring Street, New York, N.Y. 10013

Printed in the United States of America

Foreword

This volume is a continuation of the series *Critical Issues in Psychiatry: An Educational Series for Residents and Clinicians*. The series was inaugurated under the scholarly and capable editorship of Dr. Sherwyn Woods. It is appropriate to continue this series with an updated version of Dr. Horowitz's original and creative work. The earlier edition is part of the series and received wide acclaim; this book reflects the more advanced and refined thinking of Dr. Horowitz on how the psychotherapist can conceptualize and evaluate change in psychotherapy.

Dr. Horowitz continues to use the method of "configurational analysis" to describe, organize, and evaluate clinical data. He masterfully uses the case presentation method to demonstrate how to use the various stages of configurational analysis. He clearly outlines how to define problems that a patient presents and shows how to separate problems that are presented in actual sessions from those current in the patient's life and from those present from the past. He then goes on to describe how to organize the data to formulate the condition by examining patterns of verbal and nonverbal behavior. The next step in this method is to describe interpersonal behavioral patterns, self-concepts, and role relationship models; the author introduces much new information that was not previously available in this area. The fourth step describes information processing, including how to develop themes and habitual life styles. The next three steps—state, relationships, and information processing—are used to analyze process, and the final three steps describe how to examine outcome.

The reader is indebted not only to Dr. Horowitz but also to Janice, the fictitious name of a real patient. The book includes not only a detailed account of her clinical problems but also a step-by-step analysis of each of the twelve sessions with a microanalysis of her problems, as well as descriptions of the process of change in her therapy and the outcome of her therapy. The final sections of the book describe how to apply configurational analysis in teaching, in research, and in the treatment of individual patients.

The resident or practicing clinician will find a careful reading and rereading of this book invaluable in learning about the fine details of what takes place in psychotherapy, how to measure the effectiveness of the process, and how to assess outcome. The supervisor will find this book enormously helpful in teaching psychotherapy in a systematic fashion.

Dr. Horowitz is Professor of Psychiatry at the University of California in San Francisco, where he has served as the Director of the Center for the Study of Neuroses at the Langley Porter Institute. He is past president of the Northern California Psychiatric Society, the Society for Psychotherapeutic Research, and the San Francisco Psychoanalytic Institute and Society. He is recognized as a leading clinician, teacher, and researcher in psychiatry, both nationally and internationally.

Stephen C. Scheiber, M.D.

Evanston, Illinois

Preface to the Second Edition

Writing the first edition of *States of Mind* was one of the major events in my professional life. In accomplishing this task I synthesized what had been diverse modes of psychodynamic, object relations, and cognitive perspectives. The systematic approach stemming from this personal experience of containing various points of view was labeled *configurational analysis*, a term used by Erik Erikson (1954) to cover the many psychoanalytic approaches that one had to coordinate in order to understand the formation of a single dream.

With the collaboration of colleagues, the configurational analysis method was then successfully applied to new cases by teams of clinicians operating independently but viewing the same materials and utilizing the same system. Upon completion they compared views on each case studied. This led to an understanding of personality styles across various dimensions, and the variances in psychotherapy indicated by such typological differences (Horowitz, Marmar, Krupnick *et al.*, 1984). National and international interest in configurational analysis and its synthesis of cognitive and dynamic viewpoints was encouraging and gave the impetus for this second edition.

The continued input to configurational analysis has sustained the major features and elaborated certain areas of approach. Chapter 3, the formulation of maladaptive and recurrent interpersonal relationship patterns on the basis of inferences about self-concepts and role relationship models, has undergone the most revision. The changes are the result of an opportunity to establish a dialogue on person schemata between psychodynamic research clinicians and investigators from cognitive, social, and personality psychology under the auspices of the Program on Conscious and Unconscious Mental Processes initiated by the John D. and Catherine T. MacArthur Foundation. A "missing link" of theory is now added which increases the explanatory power at this step of analyzing the illustrative case material.

The illustration case is a young adult woman who was forming her adult views of self during the turbulence of reactions to a death in her family. As an immediate consequence of that death, there occurred a regressive pull to go back into the heart of her family at a time when her own progress led in other directions. Indeed, the death occurred at a crucial time when she already had unwanted states of anxiety and depression as a result of conflicts at this critical point in forming her life.

I use this case to show three main points of view that reduce previous distinctions between various brand names of theory about intrapsychic mental processes and how they may result in symptom formation or character distortions. In the first of these points, states of mind will be presented as a way to make individual personality more alive.

The other two main points will then address questions about states of mind. One point of view will focus on inner structures of meaning, especially those that summarize knowledge about self and other people. In this level of explanation, the reasons for personality consistency in different states of mind can be addressed, and the different slow and fast types of personality change can be considered. At the other level of explanation, that of how ideas and feelings are processed, it is possible to explain why, when, and how transitions occur between one state of mind and another, as well as how life events are mastered.

Mardi J. Horowitz, M.D.

San Francisco

Preface to the First Edition

Although the individuality of each of us defies any classification system, types of persons do recur. When we change, we do so in unique ways; nevertheless, repetitive patterns can be recognized. Does the behavioral scientist always have to start from ground zero when it is necessary to describe and explain a person and the change in a person? An avoidance of all theories enables him to cast the broadest possible net. But, unfortunately, he always starts at the beginning, is not alert to certain signals and so misses them, and leaves no scientific foundation upon which others can build.

On the other hand, if we approach the complexity of human personality and change with a rigid preformed theory of categories, we will make observations only according to these restrictive classifications. The scientific knowledge that we do accrue will contain distortions, and repeated observation by the same means may perpetuate these distortions. Our present belief systems contain such distortions, distortions that include illusions about those interventions that induce change processes. A proliferation of new techniques for psychotherapy marked the recent era but did not lead to a clarification of the change process; the field needs a method for careful statement of problems and examination of how, when, and why changes occurs.

Between the paths of naive empirical stances and rigid theoretical positions lies an opportune area for a flexible method of description and explanation, one whose evidence is based on observation. The configurational analysis approach described in this book is an effort at systematization of such a method. It provides a step-by-step approach to description of human problems, resources, and processes of change, and a method for assembling and organizing information. Repetition is a vital aspect of this method and results in a gradual clarification of interactive patterns; such clarification, in sequence, is essential in a complex human field wherein definitive statement by means of a single-stage analysis of evidence is impossible. The avoidance of rigid classifications or preformed definitions allows individual qualities to emerge and determine labels.

The sequence of the steps in configurational analysis begins with a summary of patterns at the level of direct observation. Inferences to explain these patterns from interactive points of view are developed gradually, at several levels of abstraction. Static situations are not predicted or necessary; the aim of the method is to describe changing situations and enduring patterns of determinants of change.

Configurational analysis is not new. It combines and expands the useful components currently inherent in our science. This is appropriate because the problems of describing persons and the changes they undergo are not new; they have been carefully studied in a variety of mental health service and research settings. Case presentations and evaluations of treatment process have been the backbone of training for all mental health professionals. But the levels of solution to the problem of how to understand, evaluate, write about, or present a given person and treatment have been so frustrating that they prompted distinguished psychologist Paul Meehl (1973) to finally write a despairing paper entitled "Why I Do Not Attend Case Conferences"!

The usual solution to the problem of organizing this kind of information goes something like this: First, there is a summary of the major problem states of the person, for instance, his episodes of suicidal rumination, anxiety attacks, or confused behavior. The person's present and past relationships to work and to significant others are then evaluated; currently active demands, conflicts, struggles, and limitations are discussed in relation to the person's controls and resources. Next, the process of treatment is explored, with focus on both the content of interaction between therapist and patient, and the form of that interaction. Finally, there is examination of outcome or current status.

Configurational analysis follows this form, but in a much more systematic manner that reduces its difficulties and prevents confusion at various levels of abstraction. Clinicians, in discussion, often do not communicate well because they focus on different parts of the total picture. The levels of abstraction most commonly confused, or even regarded as antithetical, are those of interpersonal relationship and images of self and other, and those of information processing and information control. Configurational analysis allows us to see these levels as both distinct and interactive; it allows a step-by-step look at the total picture.

One problem with the typical case conference and formulation is the multiplicity of agendas. Issues of self-esteem, conformity, and status blend with scientific objectivity. The therapist wants the patient to do well, and he wants to do well himself. Even after presentation, discussion of the issues is often cloudy. Time is short, variables are many, every discussant presents a slightly different point of view, responses are made without order, and contradictory explanations are seldom stated at similar levels of abstraction or in the same descriptive language. Much more would be gained from systematic case review by clinicians armed with an approach and with time to contemplate repeated patterns. Also, such review early in treatment would allow rational plans for subsequent interventions.

It is my hope that the main contribution of configurational analysis will be to provide a method for ordering information about a person, his problems, and the processes of change. In the material that follows, I present an outline of the steps that can lead to sequential clarification of cloudy issues, and a series of formats that can assist in the organization of information for each step. These formats are provided in two languages: linear prose and visual statement. The prose descriptions are given at the beginning of each step; the visual statements consist of diagrams that show how to organize interrelated sets of information. For example, a particular diagram about information processing shows the interrelationship between the meanings of current events, respondent ideas, enduring attitudes, emotional responses, controls, and the effect of controls on subsequent conscious experience.

The world seems to be composed of two types of people: those who are helped by diagrams and those who are confused by them. I include myself among the former and hope for some like-minded readers. For us, visual-spatial language as a complement to prose allows contemplation of ideas in two forms. I beg the forbearance of those who dislike diagrams. I have attempted to make them more palatable by using consistent formats, and have also gained confidence through teaching: Trainees who initially rejected diagrams eventually found them valuable for depicting casual interactions that might otherwise have been too cumbersome to describe clearly.

Such formats also advance a general theory of mental operations. In essence, this theory is psychoanalytic, although it modifies existing formulations. The energenic point of view is replaced by a modified ego psychology that emphasizes information processing and the structural aspects of self and object representations. Emotions are not seen as drive derivatives but as consequences of and contributors to ideation. The defense mechanisms as usually described are perceived as inadequate to explore the territory. Those classical defenses usually regarded as processes are here regarded as outcomes. Control operations are seen as the processes that accomplish these defenses. For example, undoing is viewed as the result of controls that switch sets of ideas, and so oscillate emotional or action responses; repression is seen as the result of various controls that inhibit the representation of ideas. These are not radical revisions, but efforts at increased theoretical precision. By stating controls, one in effect rotates the turret of the microscope and examines process on a finer level. This diminishes the gap between theory and clinical observation.

Configurational analysis begins with descriptions of large-scale patterns. Once they are observed, we will examine finer patterns and arrive, finally, at a microanalytic process. The systematic approach avoids a premature microanalytic preoccupation; the eventual microanalytic process is a check against the gross formations, because it compares the explanatory power of formulations with direct material such as transcripts or videotapes.

The steps of configurational analysis, and the formats for each step, are useful in training in psychopathology and psychotherapy, and in other mental health services. As a research tool, they offer a method for examining human processes of change in a repetitive manner and can be applied to successive cases selected because of similarity. They present clinicians with a means for selective case review, either to study what has happened or to plan improvements when a therapeutic impasse occurs.

Since configurational analysis lists statements in a replicable format, independent clinicians can follow this method and compare results. Wherever agreement is reached, consensual validation of patterns would be apparent. When disagreements occur, another review of the retained data would allow for adjustements to common definitions and language, or rejection of unsupported assertions. This concept of replication by use of the same format is seldom applied in clinical psychology and psychiatry, yet is is a paradigm that can encompass the richly interwoven variables of human life and the logistic and ethical problems of research with human beings.

Configurational analysis could also provide another format for organizing psychological information in applied psychodynamics. One could subject Hamlet to a description of his recurrent states of ambivalence, paralysis of action, deadly decisiveness, and pretense of gaiety or of madness; one could describe his various self-images and core models of role relationship, and explain his changes in state by the ways in which he processed information. Similarly, in a psychohistory one could plot the states, images, and information-processing styles of a person whose decisions interacted with important events.

Configurational analysis is, then, an extension of basic clinical paradigms and a movement toward greater precision and objectivity. I believe that its strength lies in its embeddedness in clinical observation, and hope that its use will advance theory and practice.

Mardi J. Horowitz, M.D.

San Francisco

Acknowledgments

Support for the research upon which this work is based was derived from the National Institute of Mental Health, through an award for six years to establish the UCSF Center for the Study of Neuroses; from the National Institute on Aging, through a grant to the Human Development Program of UCSF; and from the John D. and Catherine T. MacArthur Foundation to support the Center for the Study of Neuroses as the open-door research center of the Program on Conscious and Unconscious Mental Processes. Precursory work was supported by two Research Scientist Awards from the National Institute of Mental Health.

Charles Marmar, Nancy Wilner, Janice Krupnick, Nancy Kaltreider, Robert Wallerstein, Alan Skolnikoff, and Henry Markman worked as configurational analysts and contributed to the evolution of this method. Nancy Wilner edited the first and second editions, Jannie Dresser assisted with the second edition, and Eric Stoelting helped develop the graphic presentations.

Discussions with the faculties of UCSD, UCLA, UCD, and Stanford departments of psychiatry contributed to the configurational analysis method, as did the following individuals: Robert Rosenbaum, Katherine DeWitt, Michael Hoyt, Joseph Weiss, Harold Sampson, Emanuel Windholz, Stanley Goodman, Emmy Sylvester, Kay Blacker, Jane Loevinger, Otto Kernberg, Lorna Benjamin, Lester Luborsky, Jerome Singer, Howard Shevrin, Jacob Arlow, George Klein, Irving Janis, Richard Lazarus, David Malan, and Hans Strupp.

I am also very grateful, on behalf of all readers, to Janice, the fictional name of the person whose consent to open her therapy to research and teaching purposes permitted this contribution to be made. Other patients whose concern for the need to help others led them to make similar courageous decisions also deserve our thanks.

Contents

Introduction
Plan for Configurational Analysis: Summary of Illustration Case   1

Part I. The Definition of Problems

Chapter One
Description of Problems   21

Chapter Two
States and State Cycles   26

Chapter Three
Self-Concepts and Role Relationship Models   44

Chapter Four
Ideas, Emotions, and Controls   71

Part II. Processes of Change

Chapter Five
Modification of the Transition between States   91

Chapter Six
Development of Views of Self and Interpersonal Relationship
Patterns   96

Chapter Seven
Working Through Ideas, Feelings, and Modifying Controls   115

Part III. Description of Outcome

Chapter Eight
Alteration in the Frequency and Quality of States   145

Chapter Nine
Modification of Self-Concepts and Role Relationship Models   149

Chapter Ten
Change in Ideational Constellations and
Information-Processing Style   156

Part IV. Applications of Configurational Analysis

Chapter Eleven
Use of Configurational Analysis in Teaching   165

Chapter Twelve
Research Applications   185
(with Nancy Wilner and Charles Marmar)

Chapter Thirteen
Applications during Treatment   195

Appendices
Transcript Illustrations   207
  A. Relationship Processes: The Therapeutic Alliance   207
  B. Working Through: The Homesickness Theme   231

References   257

Index   265

)

States of Mind

Plan for Configurational Analysis: Summary of Illustration Case

This book presents a systematic method for pattern recognition in a difficult area of observation, that of human nature, individual personal problems and personality styles, and process and outcome of psychological change. This method, which is called configurational analysis, aims at clarification of psychological life. The approach is to segmentalize behavior and experience into **states** that recur; each state is then explained in terms of the schemata that organize it, and the transition of states is described in terms of how representations and expressions of meaning are regulated.

The **stability** of a given state will be explained essentially by a person's current **self-concept and inner model of relationship to others**. The **transitions** from one state to another will be examined primarily in terms of events, including internal emotions and motives and the **processing or avoidance of information** related to these events, emotions, and motives.

States, role relationships, and **information processing** are the focus of configurational analysis and they are repeatedly reviewed. The first review establishes patterns at the starting point, the second review explores patterns during change, such as in a period of therapy, and the final review examines patterns at the outcome period. These repetitions encourage gradual clarification of patterns and interactions of state relationship and information processing. Special formats for organizing information at each step of the analysis assist the overall effort. The result is exposition of the core themes that define a unique, changing personality.

Freud invented systems of classification for the purpose of describing the substructure of mental life: conscious, preconscious, and unconscious levels of mental contents; primary and secondary process modes of organizing ongoing thought; and mental functions of id, ego, and superego.

Through the concept of multiple points of view (Freud, 1923; Hartmann, 1950/1977; Rapaport and Gill, 1958; Waelder, 1930) we recognize that thought turns upon itself in complex ways so that any experience is both multidetermined and overdetermined. Unlike laboratory observations in the physical sciences, there is no single cause of an episode of human experience or behavior. While utilization of multiple points of view and the principle of overdetermination were profound gains, the language of metapsychology has been unwieldy for describing particular individual experiences. That explains Klein's (1976) differentiation of the metapsychological from the clinical psychoanalytic theory, Schafer's (1976) demand for a new language for psychoanalysis based on action concepts, Peterfreund's (1971) and Thickstun and Rosenblatt's (1977) suggested use of language based on information-processing concepts, Knapp's (1974), Gedo and Goldberg's (1973), and Greenspan and Cullander's (1973) call for new methods of case discussion and person description, and the general surge across schools for theory anchored to behavior and reportable, conscious experiences.

With recording devices, especially videotape, it is possible to make more meaningful use of that most important tool in science, repeated observation of the same data. For example, a sequence of psychotherapy can be reviewed and contemplated from multiple points of view. Repetitions assist the creative processes of pattern recognition and new combinations of concepts.

The plan for configurational analysis is to take three modes of analysis and repeat them from three points of view, with each repetition sharpening pattern description. The three modes of analysis include a description of the states of the patient, the characteristic manner of experiencing self and other during these states, and the patterns of processing or avoiding information about these interpersonal situations.

First, we will examine these modes in order to describe an illustrative patient at the onset of treatment. We will repeat this for a second time in order to understand the process of change during therapy, and for a third time in order to understand the outcome. After we have described the major patterns, we will work out the details in microanalysis of limited segments of the available data.

BACKGROUND

Anna Freud (1969), in writing on difficulties in the path of psychoanalysis, pointed out the need for plans for the organization of data about cases. Kohut (1970), in a similar inquiry into the scientific needs of psychoanalysis, stated, "The gravest danger to which analysis is exposed is the undisciplined approach of its investigators—a danger which can only be averted by preservation, in practice and in research, of the rational and orderly framework of our theory" (p. 472). The order they suggest is systematic description of cases from multiple points of view (Freud, Nagera, and Freud, 1965; Greenspan and Cullander, 1973). One sample system is the Freud *et al.* (1965) method of indexing a case by description of ego strength, nature of defenses, quality of relationships, affect expression, superego functions, drive organization, and many other factors. Another, more recent classification system, suggested by Gedo and Goldberg (1973), is one that interrelates symptomatic states, levels of cognitive structure, habitual defenses, and characteristic conflicts of a person.

Both the Freud-Nagera and Gedo-Goldberg methods are based on metapsychological terminology that is not universally accepted even in psychoanalysis. Their systems include terms based on theories still in dispute and involve high-level abstractions sometimes remote from clinical observation and the single case study. The system of configurational analysis to be described is based upon and so includes many considerations presented in these pioneering efforts but uses a less complex level of language and theoretical construction.

Knapp (1974) has also written eloquently of the need for a method for structuring the information during the study of treatment. He has suggested a naturalistic approach, one that marks off episodes according to the real flow of time, with a new segment beginning whenever a change occurs in form or content. These segments are then categorized by certain predetermined classifications. For example, the mode of experience is categorized according to the nature of experience, whether the focus is on the therapist-patient relationship, a dream, a current fantasy, introspections, reports of current life experiences, or intellectual discussion. The time frame is also defined according to whether it is immediate (the therapy session itself), current (in outside life), past, or future. Each segment can be further clarified by reducing the information, through categorizing the fantasies, emotions, and defenses that characterize it.

As with Freud–Nagera and Gedo–Goldberg, configurational analysis builds upon Knapp's conceptualizations but changes certain labels so that a more comprehensive and flexible framework is available. His episodes of emotion are placed in the general categorization of states, a term that includes felt emotion plus other aspects of experience and expression. His concept of interpersonal fantasies is included under the classification of self-image and role relationships. His category of defenses is considered, with related ideational and emotional constellations, under the more general heading of information processing.

A PLAN FOR ANALYSIS AND MICROANALYSIS

Three subheadings define the vantage points of analysis in terms of temporal perspective. The condition is defined and then formulated in terms of how the patient was **before** therapy. Then the **process** of the therapy is examined. Finally the **outcome** is considered.

These three temporal perspectives are each examined from three points of view, labeled "State," "Relationship," and "Information." **State** refers to an analysis that focuses on symptoms and signs in manifest behavior and conscious experiences. **Relationship** refers to a specific analysis of recurrent interpersonal behavioral patterns, especially those that appear as inappropriate to actual situational opportunities, and to person schemata (the key concepts of self and other that underlie and relate to states). **Information** refers to how data on self and other, and relevant environmental details, are processed by the person and includes emotional as well as intellectual expressions.

This plan is outlined in Table 1, which describes each of ten steps in condensed form. Table 2 shows the coordination of these steps by level of abstraction and temporal perspective. Ensuing chapters will describe and illustrate each step in more detail. To provide the examples each step will be applied to a specific psychotherapy so that the reader may see how steps interrelate.

No limitations of information are placed on any step. Even though the first steps formulate the condition before treatment, data from the treatment and posttreatment evaluations should be used to aid conceptualization. No clinical mystery is left for solution at the ultimate step. For this reason certain statements about outcome are made as part of the first step of problem formulation. Instead, in some instances it is useful to describe states, relationships, and informational themes "before" and "after" a change period. By looking at the differences between "before" and "after" one can designate *specific changes* and these then guide the inquiry into processes of change for the specific variables noted to change. The first steps each have an aspect of diagnostic formulation. For example, the first step indicates the presence of signs and symptoms such as hallucinations, delusions, irrational behaviors, attacks of anxiety, or phobias. The diagnostic categorizations of adjustment, neurotic, or psychotic disorders may be made during this step. The developmental diagnoses that are prominent in psychoanalytically oriented work will be a part of the formulation of core models of self and other in Step 3. For example, oedipal and preoedipal, as well as narcissistic and borderline character configurations, might be discussed in terms of the stability and fragility of self-concepts and the specific dyadic and triadic

Table 1. The Ten Steps of Configurational Analysis

Defining the Condition

Step 1. *Problems:* List symptoms, signs, and problems. Separate the initial complaints made by the patient from problems reported subsequently; also list difficulties the observer recognizes but the patient does not complain of directly, indicating the evidence for these inferences.

Include both intrusions and omissions from rational consciousness and behavior. Intrusions are episodes of consciousness or action that are unwanted, unbidden, or hard to dispel, such as an impending sense of doom, an unwelcome repetition in memory, images of a traumatic event, or a temper outburst. Omissions include the absence of desired and adaptive experiences or actions, such as inability to become sexually aroused, inability to recollect a loved one, and failures to confront the implications of important situations. Separate these classes of symptoms and signs into those current in the actual sessions, those current in life outside the session, and those that were present in the past.

Make diagnoses based on signs and symptoms as they combine into syndromes and disorders at this point.

Formulating the Condition

Step 2. *State:* List recurrent states and define them by patterns of verbal and nonverbal behavior, as well as by reports of subjective experiences. Indicate common shifts between states, frequency and duration of any given state, and triggers for entry into problematic states.

Begin with states that contain the major symptomatic phenomena described in Step 1. After listing the major symptomatic state, usually in the undermodulated category, list other undermodulated states. Next list states that seem more controlled. Complete the list with overcontrolled states of mind. Discuss these states according to their motivational and defensive arrangements: which states are desired, dreaded, which states are compromises that reduce pleasure but prevent risk of displeasurable states.

Step 3. *Interpersonal behavioral patterns, self-concepts, and role relationship models:* Describe the recurrent maladaptive interpersonal behavioral patterns that are related to the problems as defined as Steps 1 and 2. Then infer and describe the intrapsychic person schemata, motives, and personal agendas upon which these maladaptive patterns are based. When there is sufficient information, reconstruct the probable development of the views contained in these schemata.

A. Repetoire of self- and object schemata: List the self- and object concepts of the person, and describe his or her highest developmental achievement in terms of integrating these into supraordinate views.

B. Role relationship models: Organize the self- and object view into models that suggest complementarity in aims and expectations of response. Relate each state in Step 2 to these role relationship models, attempting to posit the main model for a given state.

C. Scripts, schematic agendas, and story lines: Describe schematic sequences of role relationship models as they are inferred to underlie repetitive maladaptive interpersonal patterns.

(Continued)

Table 1. (*Continued*)

Formulating the Condition (*Continued*)

D. *Relationship conflicts.* Model conflicts and/or deficiencies surrounding the personal agenda of the individual at the present life development period. Include regressive as well as progressive aims. Describe how recent life events may have activated latent conflictual relationship themes or warded off self-concepts.

Step 4.　*Information processing:* As a point of departure, take from the problem list repetitive intrusions and omissions from rational consciousness. Model central themes of conflict as constellations of ideas, emotions, and maneuvers of control over modes of representing and communicating thought and feeling. Include wishes, threats, and defenses.

A. *Themes*

(1) Indicate major constellations of memories and fantasies as composites of ideas, feelings, and actions that influence current states of mind, especially those related to the problem states described in Step 2. Describe trains of thought that are initiated by wishes or needs and that activate the problematic self- and object concepts described in Step 3. Relate these constellations to recent life events, physiological conditions, and social situations.

(2) Derive a model of the degree to which outer reality accords with the subject's conscious views, assumptions, and unconscious organizing schematizations. Indicate how discrepancies between outer world and inner assumptions, or between inner motives and inner critical or moral assessments, evoke emotional responses and lead the subject to control efforts that may lead to coping strategies, defensive maneuvers, or failures to cope well.

(3) Derive a model of how control operations influence the processing of themes consciously and unconsciously.

(4) If information is available, indicate why progression toward completion of a train of thought, emotional working through, or decision making is blocked for each theme, noting the developmental basis for the wishes, threats, and defenses involved.

B. *Habitual styles:* Indicate the subject's typical use of modes of representation and information-processing strategies and how this leads to habitual defensive operations, or character traits. Relate different modes for processing or representing information to different states of mind noted in Step 2.

Analysis of Process: Develop Explanatory Statements for Recurrent Patterns in Therapeutic Process

Step 5.　*State:* Review entry into and exit from the states listed in Step 2 as they occur in therapy or are reported for current outside-of-session relationships. Divide the therapy or time of change into phases according to times of transition in state patterns, such as changes in typical state occurrences or cycles. When indicated, describe the states of the therapist or therapist and patient as a pair or small group. Describe the effect of interventions on the transitions between states. Include the effect of new external events on states and continuation of process after therapy when such data are available. If medication has been used, describe changes in states in relation to the time of use of the pharmaceutical agents. Include description of economic, environmental, or social situational changes.

Table 1. (*Continued*)

Analysis of Process (*Continued*)

Step 6. *Relationships:* For each phase of therapy described in Step 5 describe changes in interpersonal relationships and self-concepts. Use the labels for self and other roles defined in Step 3. Discuss separations and new attachments. Then discuss the various relationships of the patient with the therapist, including social alliances, therapeutic alliances, transferences, and countertransferences. Indicate dilemmas of the therapist caused by alternative relationship views by the patient. The sequence of tests by the patient for relationship potentials, and the therapist's manner of dealing with these issues, can be summarized. Discuss actual and potential errors of technique provoked by the patient or made by the therapist. Describe useful and unhelpful techniques for dealing with relationship issues.

Step 7. *Information processing:* Classify interventions by the therapist in relation to key themes and defensive resistances as outlined for constellations of ideas, emotions, and defenses. Describe the focus of attention and levels of interpretation used by the therapist. Focus on work (or failure to work) on the main themes and defensive styles described in Step 4, on explanations of the shifting state patterns in different phases of therapy described in Step 5, and on explanation of the processes of changing relationship patterns described in Step 6. Describe how therapist interventions affected the patient's control processes and explain changes in the patient's key attitudes, beliefs, and ability to plan or restrain intended actions.

Examination of Outcome

Step 8. *States:* Describes outcome in terms of changes in signs, symptoms, and states. Include discussion of interaction of situational factors with change, including family, social, environmental, and neurobiological systems. Discuss new states, state cycles, and state triggers. Use labels from Steps 2 and 5.

Step 9. *Interpersonal behavioral patterns, self-concepts, and role relationship models:* Describe the outcome in terms of changes and persistences of maladaptive interpersonal behavioral patterns and patterns of self-regard. Include an analysis of changes in personal contacts, family, social structure, and situational opportunities that may have played a role in the changes noted. Infer the changes and developments in person schemata that may have led to these alterations in behavior. Include modifications in enduring attitudes, value hierarchies, and personal agendas.

Step 10. *Information processing*

A. *Themes:* Describe outcome in terms of changes or shifts in the themes described in Step 4. Relate these modifications to changes in emotional responses, memories, and fantasies. Include comments about increased or decreased scope of life purposes or plans.

B. *Habitual styles:* Describe changes in coping, defensive, or conceptual styles noted in Steps 4 and 7.

Table 2. Outline of the Sequence of Steps

Defining the condition Step 1	Pretherapy condition	Change process	Outcome condition
States	Step 2	Step 5	Step 8
Relationship	Step 3	Step 6	Step 9
Information	Step 4	Step 7	Step 10

relationship problems of the given patient. Finally, personality styles will be described again in the form of statements about information processing, coping, and the defensive maneuvers (Step 4).

External situational factors are considered in each step. Events and environmental contexts will be included in discussion of problems; onset of a symptom, for example, will be placed in temporal relationship to precipitating stresses such as the loss of a loved one. Events will also be included in states, as they effect changes in state. Similarly, the entry, exit, and action of significant persons, as well as other happenings, will be incorporated into relationship analyses. Any event, including actions of the self, will be treated as information in that section, in terms of news that is recognized, interpreted, and used in problem solving and decision making.

ILLUSTRATION CASE

In order to maintain coherence of set across description of the steps of configurational analysis, a single case provides the material for these examples. A brief therapy of 12 hours is used to show that configurational analysis does not necessarily require extensive data. Indeed, it can even be used to organize information from a single interview or fragment.

Janice, the name we will use to designate the patient, is in her mid-twenties. She gave informed consent to the recording of the interviews and to the use of these materials for teaching and research purposes. Selected verbatim transcripts, with deletion or changing of real names and places will illustrate key points. No special technique makes the therapy dramatic; in that sense, the reader will review an ordinary psychotherapy. There was a more than average difficulty in establishing a therapeutic focus for this brief therapy, and examination of this difficulty is useful in showing how complex processes can be illuminated by configurational analysis. Janice's unusual intelligence and articulateness gives expressive clarity to these transcripts.

Because of a research context for the therapy, there were rating scales, and evaluation and follow-up interviews were conducted by an independent clinician. Since recordings of all interviews were video- as well as audiotaped, the material available included complete transcripts, process notes, summaries by the evaluator and therapist, and rating scales by the patient, evaluator, and therapist.

Identifying Information and Referral

Janice is a twenty-four-year-old woman with a college degree that she received several months before her clinic entry. She lived with a boyfriend and had a position as an assistant group worker. She called the psychiatric clinic less than two weeks after returning from a funeral for her younger brother, who had died suddenly and unexpectedly. She felt unable to mourn, feared she might "fall apart," and was "unable to get herself together."

Stress Event and Other Presenting Complaints

When she came home from work one day, Janice was informed that her brother had died. She felt initial disbelief and countered it by saying, "But it can't be a joke." Then she immediately focused her attention on practical arrangements, such as a reservation for the plane trip to her home. "Right away, I started avoiding it, cried only a little, and shifted to an intellectual plane to ward off tears." Additional self-imposed controls took the form of distancing through self-observation and dramatization. She noted in herself a condescending quality toward any expression of emotions.

In addition to "inability to openly mourn his loss" and the fear that she might "fall apart" she told the evaluator of her concern that her responses might interfere with her performance on her recently acquired job. She reported that reminders of her brother triggered intrusive thoughts about the death. She had a few nightmares related to death, and dreams of her family that she could not recall. Otherwise she had "floating thoughts" about her relationship with her dead brother "with no feelings attached." She had been worried by fantasies that her boyfriend might die.

She also described periodic depressions present before the death, in which she felt lazy and sulky, and characterized these depressions as "getting in touch with the real me," and as related to onset of monthly menses and to feelings of "constantly failing" in relationships with men and her mother. She managed these depressions by withdrawal, by retreating to her bed, "indulging" herself in amusements that required "no thought," since at such times "any thought is dangerous." Since arriving locally, she had one telephone contact with a treatment resource, around feelings related to depression over her "low achievement," but did not follow through as she "never quite had the time."

Additional Responses Related to the Death

Additional information emerged only late in the course of therapy but is presented here in the usual case summary form. The vague circumstances surrounding the death contributed to a sense of unreality about the event. Additional fantasies developing around the event were in the form of denial, such as "the CIA rigged the death and are now using him as an undercover agent." Such fantasies had no basis in reality, and no sense, to her, of being real.

Her feelings were heightened and confused at the funeral, one week later. Janice had returned to her home for the services and to spend two weeks with her family, but the funeral engendered much family conflict. She and her younger siblings, for she was the oldest, treated the services as a "celebration of his life"; the younger generation was angered with efforts by the family to "turn it into a funeral." The patient served as a "leader against family solidarity" around the issue of how to hold the funeral. She was criticized by her mother for "fooling around and being silly."

At home, prior to the funeral, Janice avoided visitors who came to console the family. She withdrew upstairs to rest on her bed and avoid confrontation with her mother's tears and the "special attention" her mother received from comforting friends. She alternated between feelings of disgust for her mother's emotional display, and admiration for her mother's ability to cry and not "stay in bed." This brother had been Janice's favorite sibling because he especially admired and praised her rebellious independence and leadership during adolescence. Nonetheless she felt "my role wasn't chief mourner, by any means; that was mother's role."

She was, as mentioned, criticized for "acting weird" and felt quite vulnerable to criticism because she did not cry at the funeral and withdrew upstairs when consoling friends and relatives came to the house. She also felt angry, disgusted, and in opposition to perceived "expectations" of her behavior. "I was a square peg in a round hole." She felt she maintained her separation and distance from the family through not "succumbing" ("getting sucked in") to the funeral tradition of tears, even in the face of her mother's plea that "this is **not** the time to be independent . . . at least **now**, behave yourself." She had feelings of wanting "unqualified" love from her mother at the funeral and conflicted flight and irritation responses when her mother urged her to "now" stay at home with the family and, in effect, end her independence.

Past History

The patient is the oldest of several surviving siblings raised in an intact, middle-class, mainstream American family. Her father is described as stable and caring, but unable to express emotion. He felt successful in his work as a union officer, always emphasized his high expectations that Janice obtain good grades, engage in important activities, and achieve "golden" popularity. She saw her mother as a constant and committed housewife and mother who married at an early age, and, somewhat disappointed, looked for gratification through raising her children, whom she loved. At this time she felt her mother had shown "qualified" and conditional love, "**saying** I want you to be happy, but **meaning** I want you to be what I want you to be."

She saw her parents' relationship as interlocking, supportive, but also quietly conflictual. The mother turned to the patient as a "confidante" and expressed her feelings of sexual frustration and low self-esteem. She always cared for the children while her husband took many side trips for the union, with no consideration of a vacation for her. She "submitted" to her husband's expectations and felt unable to leave the children in his care, even temporarily. She was overweight because she turned to food for comfort, a pattern she fostered in her children. She felt her life was "lost," that she should never have married him. Janice felt pushed by her mother to make the same choices: "I have to live **her** life to prove it was worth **her** having done it."

Although denying sibling rivalry, the patient always felt "special." She was the oldest, and "the only girl for a long time," and was only a little over a year old when the next sibling was born. She felt some guilt in relation to always "outshining" this next-younger brother. She globally recalls a "happy, happy childhood." Play with girl friends alternated with withdrawal to solitary reading. Her father would then tease and admonish her to "go out and play . . . you do **everything** reading a book."

The patient and her siblings were characterized as "rebellious . . . we've all given them [parents] as much trouble as we could." The patient recalls various restrictions placed on her during adolescence. She was prohibited from going barefoot to high school because such behavior would reflect on her mother, who would be seen in the community as a "bad mother."

Janice had a particular conflict with her parents around her sexuality and their strict, religious, and conventional morality. As soon as her mother discovered that she engaged in and enjoyed sexual relationships, "we've been fighting in that area ever since," with her mother alternately stating that women could not enjoy sexual relationships until marriage, predicting sexual failure altogether, or accusing the patient of being a "nymphomaniac or a slut."

Janice had an early school history characterized by high academic achievement. She was told that she had high IQ scores by her teachers, who suggested relative underachievement, "a lot of potential I never lived up to." It was thought that here relatively high academic performance was interfered with by difficulties in interpersonal relationships. For example, she was on academic probation for a time immediately following a breakup with a lover. She completed college while living at home, and after graduation moved away in order to become independent.

Work experience since her local arrival had a quality of "underemployment." She held clerical positions briefly and then took her present job, characterized as "flunky's work." Her work conflicts emerged in the form of a "bad attitude": She was criticized for working slowly and too casually, was irritated at feeling unappreciated, and excused herself and solicited attention through somatic complaints. While dissatisfied, she also felt that her current job at a home for the elderly was "safe . . . not too challenging."

Although initially insistent about the absence of any "homesickness" for family or friends, she later acknowledged that "functioning on her own" during the past year had been difficult, recalling that during an earlier separation while in college, she missed her family. Family pressures to return home continued and she resisted, feeling unable to do so until she had developed her own "self," "so I can stand up to her [mother]." Her stated future plans were that she would return to school for an advanced degree with an ultimate wish to marry (in the abstract) "for the title, legitimacy, and status."

Aside from Phillip, with whom she had lived for the past three months, Janice had few friends in this area and only one close woman friend in another part of the country. Her feelings remained "foggy" concerning Phillip. Her previous boyfriend was "intellectual, verbal, and dazzled me." Phillip was described as sensitive and attractive, although he was nonverbal, not college-educated, and had reading difficulties, but "has **thought** about things a lot and pays attention to **me**." She saw him as similar to her father, in that he was sometimes unresponsive to her. She found this frustrating. "It makes me feel worthless." While considering the relationship "in flux . . . not an established thing," she suspected that she was "using him for security . . . the one-room apartment is like a womb . . . he accepts me." Before coming to therapy she had begun to feel she ought to break up with him.

Since the death of her brother, the patient had feared losing Phillip, likening him to an "underdog" (as was her brother). At one point she had a fantasy of Phillip's death through "brain disease," and imagined herself crying at **his** funeral. In that fantasy the funeral was also attended by his ex-woman friend competing for the position of "chief mourner" (similar to feelings related to her mother at her brother's funeral). Such fantasies were associated with fears of being alone and "vegetating," feeling that she might be unable to establish new relationships due to her perceived tendency to "suck everything out of relationships . . . demand and demand until the poor guy breaks," and drawing parallels with "a friend" who is in a "bad relationship out of fear of not getting anyone else."

Past Therapy

The patient's first therapeutic contact, when a senior in high school, was through counseling around conflicts related to "loss of her virginity." She again sought help as a college freshman after she "fell apart" following the end of a one-year relationship and "missed the whole spring" of that academic year.

Attitude to Present Therapy

Initial expectations and fears regarding therapy were that her previously perceived "introspection and self-awareness" was "all talk," and that she would be unable to "feel" in therapy, would impress the therapist with her intelligence and abilities, and would be unable to get in touch with and resolve her depressive feelings. Perceived therapeutic risks involved fear of loss of the relationship with Phillip once she "looked at it clearly," fear that therapy would make her "worse," questioning whether she **really** wanted to experience "the feelings," and fears that she would become even more introspective or dependent.

Self-Description

The patient stated that she had always wanted to be a composer, should have written her first sonata by the age of seventeen, felt that it was already "too late," was a "snob about status," and "should be a symphony conductor." (Although she procrastinated whenever she thought of practicing or composing music.) In addition to underachieving and "fearing failure," she viewed herself as never experiencing authentic feelings, as "acting" open while being secretive, as behaving like a "modern woman" while feeling like "giving up" and becoming an asexual old lady. Her body image, sometimes, was that she was "fat-ugly-disgusting." She felt she had no "will power," preferring to "control things" to the extent of knowing "about things before they happen." Interpersonal relationships were colored by her feeling that she was greedy (to the extent of referring to herself as a "vampire"), and by her efforts to manipulate others to compliment her or feel sorry for her. If she was successful at getting pity she felt contempt for the person fooled into offering it. She felt like a failure when relationships ended but entered them with the covert statement "Here I am, totally worthless, love me anyway, and I'll think less of you if you do."

Initial Objective Description of the Patient

The patient was casually dressed, attractive, slightly overweight. She communicated by using many facial expressions and hand movements for additional dramatic emphasis, but maintained a fixed smile; beneath it she seemed affectively flat. Her voice was high-pitched, sometimes strained with lapses into sounding childlike or wistful, especially when talking of her mother. She spoke abstractly or about peripheral details when questioned by the interviewer. She seemed to deliberately keep emotional ideas at a distance by vagueness, denial, intellectualization, and shifting between topics or shifting between personal stances on topics.

Brief Review of the Treatment

Janice began the evaluation interview by talking about the death of her brother. She couldn't believe it, and tended to intellectualize it or avoid thinking about it altogether. She also reported feeling periodically depressed, even before the death of her brother. She had concerns about discovering the "real me." She seemed eager to obtain therapy, although she indicated a fear of dramatizing herself and a fear of feeling too sad. Logistic arrangements for the once-a-week, time-limited brief therapy were easily settled.

The **first therapy interview** meant introduction to another clinician. She presented herself as articulate and at ease, but seemed tense underneath. She repeated the story about her brother's death, told of anger at various authority figures involved in the death and postdeath period. She said she tended to use news of the event mainly to get sympathy, and was not experiencing the sadness that she thought was deep within her. The therapist felt there was a diffusion of focus and that she struggled against his aims to establish a focus. In his process note he predicted emergence in the treatment relationship of aims for independence in conflict with wishes to remain attached to parental figures. He thought competitive struggles with him would emerge as a theme and noted a warded-off, dull, blunted type of depression.

The **second interview** focused on her resistances to treatment, especially her need to avoid being degraded by exposure. The therapist observed that she was using several filters to separate herself from the ideas she communicated. As an intervention, he asked her to recollect and imagine aspects of the death of her brother. There was no emotional response. But she came close to tears later in the hour when the therapist said that now that she had left home, she was on new paths in her life that would lead her toward that which she wished to become. After this intervention, she said she was yearning for friendship with a woman.

At the beginning of the **third interview** she seemed more pressured, but tried a jolly manner. The interview focused on her relationship with her parents, especially their criticism of her behavior. Her father was more overtly critical; he had told her she was stupid for living with a person like Phillip. Her mother, while basically more covert in her criticism, had accused Janice of being a nymphomaniac and urged her to be more like **she** was. Other interview contents were related to the death of her brother, with some reference to the funeral and a hint of unsatisfactory events, but no details. A new complaint emerged about how she was close to being fired from her work because of difficulties with her supervisor.

The therapist's main interventions concerned her fears of therapy. Otherwise he sought clarification of the relationship with her parents since that was where her affect and defensiveness led. There was some focus on the therapy itself, on how the goals seemed diffuse. The use of the story about her brother's death was seen as a ticket of admission to therapy she wanted for other unclarified reasons.

In the **fourth interview**, there was some discussion of an hour she had missed the previous week because it occurred on her birthday and she had been depressed. She had stayed home crying. She said she called to cancel, but no message was left for the therapist. In this session she was more depressed than in any previous session and seemed to verge on quitting. Content revolved around how she was treated unfairly at the home for the elderly where she worked and so felt herself to be the lowest person there. The therapist pointed out that she provoked the criticism by behaving at work in a passive-aggressive manner. When she felt hurt by this, the therapist said she was angry and depressed by his remark, and she was able to acknowledge that this was so.

She seemed more relaxed in the **fifth interview**, at about the same level as in the first interviews. The hour focused on the issue of establishing a therapeutic contract. The agreed-upon aim, developed after considerable struggle in which she wanted the therapist to agree to give her "an acceptable image of herself," was to focus on her feelings of herself as bad, disgusting, or defective. There was some further work on recognition of the passive-aggressive patterns that provoked the criticism that frightened her about losing her job.

In the **sixth interview**, she used a stomachache to get attention from the therapist. She talked about Phillip and how she would like to get away from him if she could only bear the thought of being alone. She tested the therapist to see how much he would do for her and wavered between disclosing more of herself and trying to present a superficially good picture. The therapist listened during most of the hour, making an occasional intervention to link her difficulties with Phillip to her bad self-images. In his process notes he remarked that he felt they were diffusing again without much work accomplished.

In the **seventh interview**, Janice asked the therapist to review the goals of therapy that had been set in the previous hours. This was seen as a struggle with the therapist that, in the course of its resolution, strengthened the working relationship. She then reported a dream of the dead brother that she had the night before this interview. In that dream he told her not to miss him because she still had other siblings.

In the **eighth interview**, she indicated she had had turbulent feelings since the previous interview, including crying for a whole day, but had felt better as the present interview approached. She indicated improvement in her ability to avoid excessive eating and withdrawal from contact with others. She talked of how she cried or used the story about the brother's death to get sympathy. The therapist then centered on how she had only recently left her family, was uncommitted to a future plan, and so felt homesick. The patient and therapist then discussed how the funeral had intensified her wish to return home. She had always felt a pull to be like her mother, and yet had an even stronger wish to separate herself and find her own roles. A much greater feeling of cooperation and alliance was developed. Interventions linked her search for attachment with feelings of frustration, and the contempt and hostility she felt when her wishes were not gratified.

In the **ninth interview** she came prepared to talk about bad images of herself in relation to her living partner. The therapist listened for a long time and then confronted her with her vagueness and distance from him. The hour then focused on her difficulties in adjustment during this year of being away from her family, and the relationship of the funeral to her struggle over whether to return or escape from the influence of her parents.

She began the **tenth interview** by saying she had been feeling better and more optimistic. She had gone to see an aunt and while with her felt, for the first time, a sense of mutual mourning in response to the death of her brother. She talked clearly for the first time about how inappropriate her behavior at the funeral had been, describing silly activities and withdrawal when she should have been mourning with her relatives. The therapist aimed at clarifying her feelings of guilt because she had not had authentic feelings, her feelings of anger with her mother during the funeral for both establishing and not reestablishing a child-parent relationship, and for her mother's use of the occasion to seek sympathy for herself.

In the **eleventh interview**, she appeared amiable and in good control. She reviewed material discussed in the previous hour and focused on her relationship with her mother. The therapist narrowed this down further by helping her to a detailed reconstruction of interactions with her mother during the funeral, and of how this mirrored long-standing conflicts. An ambivalent but close—even partially merged—attachment between Janice and her mother was the topic of most interpretations. The relationship of these themes to impending termination was discussed, as was the idea of engaging in treatment for characterological problems at a later time.

Janice seemed poised and businesslike at the **final interview**, more distant from the therapist than during hours 8–11. She decided not to seek further treatment, because she wanted to be independent and see how things fit together for herself. She generally reviewed main themes. There was agreement that there had been a good therapeutic outcome.

Follow-up

Janice returned two months after termination of treatment for a posttherapy **evaluation interview** with the same clinician she had seen before treatment. She reported a general feeling of being more positive in her view of herself. She had been less depressed, less withdrawn, and had improved her work. She felt the therapy had been very helpful and had a good memory for what had happened during it. Her relationship with Phillip was still at issue and related to her wish not to seek further therapy: She feared that it might result in the ending of what appeared to be a dependent relationship. She felt she was more realistic in relation to her brother's death and gave evidence that she was in the midst of a gradual mourning response.

A **second posttherapy evaluation interview** was conducted ten months after the termination of the treatment. She described positive changes in her life. She had a clear feeling of increased control and a positive self-concept. Depressive episodes remained less frequent and more attenuated than before treatment. She had continued to improve her work and had been praised and rewarded. In addition, she had made plans for advanced education. She had separated amicably from Phillip and was living more independently, seeing him occasionally. She felt good about her decreased dependence upon others and had renewed a close relationship with a female friend. She also felt increasingly adult in her relationship to her parents, and planned to join them in a family reunion, during which they would scatter the ashes of her brother. She had decided to seek additional therapy, but chose group therapy because she wanted to maintain her sense of independence from any one authority. She expressed positive feelings about the benefits of therapy and the therapist.

SUMMARY

Configurational analysis is a system that aims at sequential steps for the clarification of processes of change. Three time perspectives are involved, covering the period before and after a change as well as the time of change. For each time perspective, states, relationships, and information-processing patterns are examined. The repetition from altered points of view helps both the shape of pattern description and the examination of interactive effects. Background case material has been given and will be developed as an illustration of this method.

I

The Definition of Problems

CHAPTER ONE

Description of Problems

Defining The Condition

Step 1. Problems: *List symptoms, signs, and problems. Separate the initial complaints made by the patient from problems reported subsequently; also list difficulties the observer recognizes but the patient does not complain of directly, indicating the evidence for these inferences.*

Include both intrusions and omissions from rational consciousness and behavior. Intrusions are episodes of consciousness or action that are unwanted, unbidden, or hard to dispel, such as an impending sense of doom, an unwelcome repetition in memory, images of a traumatic event, or a temper outburst. Omissions include the absence of desired and adaptive experiences or actions, such as inability to become sexually aroused, inability to recollect a loved one, and failures to confront the implications of important situations. Separate these classes of symptoms and signs into those current in the actual sessions, those current in life outside the session, and those that were present in the past.

Make diagnoses based on signs and symptoms as they combine into syndromes and disorders at this point.

Human psychology, because of its subjectivity and complexity, makes problem statement more difficult than statement of physical infirmities. Initially, the person may only admit to certain problems and hold back others because of embarrassment. Some problems may not be immediately known and emerge later, perhaps as new awareness during a treatment process. Finally, one person evaluating another may appraise some issues as problems, without agreement of the subject.

The configurational analysis format segregates themes on the problem list according to **who** knows about the problem during the period defined as a starting point, such as a first clinical evaluation. The format also suggests statement of the status of that problem for the outcome period after the change process under consideration has taken place. This gives any reviewer an immediate overview of what has happened. A problem list can begin when only pretherapy information is available. It will help the clinician maintain clarity on initial issues and supply a baseline for noting changes.

A first heading on the problem list should classify the initial problems stated by the patient, segregated into **specific** and **general** complaints. A subheading covers **additional complaints**, in some instances reported after the initial interview. It may be useful to subdivide this section further into problems concerned with self-regard, and problems viewed in terms of relationships with others. Finally, there should be room for problems formulated from observation by the **clinician**.

Illustration

The problem list for Janice is shown in Table 3. Since Janice was seen in an investigative as well as a therapeutic context, quantitative measures of distress are available to illustrate how such data can be related to problems as they are clinically described. Such means on general scales are much less specific than an individualized problem statement but, when examined in conjunction with such statements, can convey degree of distress, magnitude of change, and relationship of information about the particular patient to averages derived from other patients.

A relevant example is the self-report of Janice as she completed the Hopkins Symptom Checklist (Derogatis, Lipman, and Covi, 1973), checking off 90 symptoms (such as "feeling lonely") on a five-point scale from zero (not at all) to four (extremely). The SCL-90 can be repeated, as it was with Janice, yielding scores for periods before and after therapy. Subscales for somatization, obsessive-compulsive items, interpersonal sensitivity, depression, anxiety, anger-hostility, phobic anxiety, paranoid ideation, and psychoticism have been established. Her highest scores at the pretherapy period were on the depression and obsessive-compulsion subscales. A graphic display of the scores on these scales, as well as her overall symptomatic level, indicates that there was a reduction in these main symptom patterns during the therapy, that the

Table 3. Problem List

Before therapy	Status after therapy
Complaints (Initially made by patient)	
1. *Specific:* not grieving properly for her brother who recently died	Grieving
2. *General:* several years of "depressions" characterized by apathy, withdrawal, feeling foggy and unreal, overeating, feelings of self-digust	Less depressed, less foggy, more real; more goal-directed behavior, less self-disgust; still overeating; no new symptoms
Additional Problems (Emerged from patient during early therapy hours)	
1. *Problems with self:* episodically unable to motivate self to work, leading to fear of losing job	Able to do better work, seeking advanced education
2. *Problems with others:* sometimes too competitive, negative, passive-aggresive, dependent, dramatic, or pretending	Some improvement in dependency, pretending, negativism. Unchanged competitive and dramatic traits
3. Remorseful over behavior at brother's funeral	Accepts, understandingly, that she did not cry at brother's funeral
Formulated Problems (Inferences by therapist)	
1. Negative and defective self-images defended against by role playing of positive self-images	Increase in self-esteem with stabilization of more positive self-images, still vulnerable to deflation of self-regard
2. Unresolved attachment to mother with ambivalent identification. Aims for independence in conflict with wish for dependence, and fear of hurting mother by detachment. Subordination-domination struggles result	Improved sense of independence from mother with residual conflicts and subordination-domination struggles
3. Incomplete mourning with denial of affect and with strong component of narcissistic injury due to loss	Mourning process underway, not completed. Able to experience pangs of sadness and anger with sense of self-control

symptoms continued to abate in the posttreatment period, and that improvement was fairly well maintained over the ensuing year (see Figure 1).

Concordant findings occur on examination of clinician rating scales done by both the evaluator and the therapist. The Brief Psychiatric Rating Scale (Overall and Gorham, 1962) contains eight neurotic dysfunction scales, including one for the depressive mode. They were rated at every

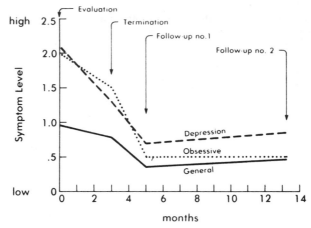

Figure 1. Levels of the Highest Symptom Subsets and General Symptom Level over Time According to Repeated Patient Reports on Symptom Checklist (SCL-90).

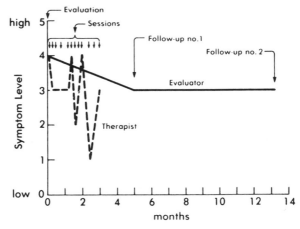

Figure 2. Levels of Depression over Time as Rated by Evaluator and Therapist on Brief Psychiatric Rating Scale.

encounter and the depression subscale again yielded one of the highest scores.

The evaluator and therapist agreed with the patient in that they also rated her depressive mood as decreasing with treatment (see Figure 2). Overall symptoms, from eight other subscales, also declined in a similar manner (see Figure 3).

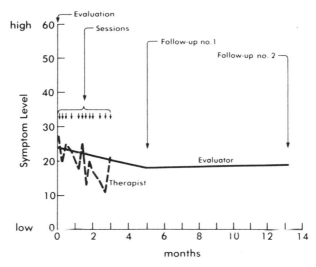

Figure 3. General Symptom Level over Time as Rated by Evaluator and Therapist on Brief Psychiatric Rating Scale.

Diagnosis

As mentioned earlier, diagnostic formulations allow professionals to communicate rapidly and to relate a specific case to agreed-upon abstractions and general implications. If one used the current official nomenclature of the American Psychiatric Association (1980, at this writing), Janice would have been diagnosed as having an "Adjustment Disorder of Adult Life," specifically, a pathological grief reaction. This would be an Axis I diagnosis. As for Axis II, on personality diagnosis Janice did not fit perfectly into any category. She had some hysterical and obsessional personality qualities and a degree of narcissistic traits, but few if any paranoid, schizoid, or borderline character traits.

SUMMARY

Problem lists that show conditions before and after a change process provide conceptual anchors for the discussion of change. In attempting such clarification, it is useful to separate descriptions that are focal and specific from those that are global and general, and to designate who defines a given behavior or experience as a problem.

CHAPTER TWO

States and State Cycles

Formulating the Condition

Step 2. State: List recurrent states and define them by patterns of verbal and nonverbal behavior, as well as by reports of subjective experiences. Indicate common shifts between states, frequency and duration of any given state, and triggers for entry into problematic states.

Begin with states that contain the major symptomatic phenomena described in Step 1. After listing the major symptomatic state, usually in the undermodulated category, list other undermodulated states. Next list states that seem more controlled. Complete the list with overcontrolled states of mind. Discuss these states according to their motivational and defensive arrangements: which states are desired, dreaded, which states are compromises that reduce pleasure but prevent risk of displeasurable states.

State description is a way of condensing multiple observations into a limited set of patterns. Since any person can exhibit or report multiple states of behavior and experience, a selective process operates in establishing a relevant list of states. Relevance is defined by the particular context, the specific person, and the time span under consideration. The problem states provide a usual point of departure.

Unlike diagnostic statements, state descriptions go beyond generalities to individual nuances of experience and behavior. Labels such as "panicky emptiness" are elaborated to include the way a particular person senses and displays such fear. Moreover, the matrix of problem states of the person includes other common and recurrent states. A model of the frequent state transitions is then developed. The description of states and the patterns of state transition provide a powerful technique for defining the surface characteristic of a given individual personality at a given period. One can then move on to an explanation of the stability of a given state; to understanding why if it is painful or maladaptive it continues and repeatedly recurs.

A DEFINITION OF STATES

A state has already been described as a recurrent pattern of experience and of behavior that is both verbal and nonverbal. States are commonly recognized during a clinical interview because of changes in facial expression, intonation and inflection in speech, focus and content of verbal reports, degree of self-reflective awareness, general arousal, shifts in degree and nature of empathy, and other communicative qualities. The information that tells the observer, or the subject, that this is a recurrence of a familiar state is not confined to any one system but is a configuration of information in multiple systems.

The states of a particular person are as easy to recognize in everyday life as the change of atmosphere in a drama, from cheerful sunlight to thunder and lightning, the shifts of configuration in rhythm, harmony, timber, and tonality in music, or the mood of color, hue, texture, form, and content in a painting. A state description may include, for behavioral form, the patterns noted in posture, facial expression, tone of voice, gestures, style of speech flow, dialect, deployment of gaze, and other physical signs of attention focus. These will often convey the emotional coloration of a given state of mind. For verbal report, the specific thought contents, felt emotions as labeled in words or described in images of bodily feelings, and other reported aspects of subjective experience may be included. The congruence between verbal and nonverbal is also of interest, especially as emotional colorations are considered. Some states are prominent in having a discrepancy between the type of mood conveyed in physical expressions and that reported verbally. In addition, the feeling of the observer for the subject's degree of apparent volitional control over expressions and actions is often useful as an aspect of state description. The triggers of entry into that state and the instigators of exiting from that state complete a good state description.

By labeling a state one derives a name for a kind of experience. This label then suffices to refer to all the patterns that cohere to form a state of mind. A name also allows better conscious contemplation of states, so that additional observation can be made. A dictionary of state terms may help derive such names. One organized by major emotional colorations is found at the end of this chapter (see Table 6).

Each person has many states. State analysis requires selection of those that are most relevant. It also means that the natural flow of behavior and experience must be somewhat artificially segmented into episodes defined by differences in quality.

Background

The earliest clinical state descriptions involved severe psychopathology, since the social relevance of recurrent episodes of irrational behavior compelled careful observation. Transient periods of delusional behavior, anxiety attacks, and multiple personalities in a single individual provided early impetus for state analyses (Gaarter, 1971).

Dissociative states were described for four thousand years as prominent symptoms of hysterical psychoneuroses (Vieth, 1977). These syndromes were explored in depth and explained in terms of unconscious roles, aims, fears, and defenses by Breuer and Freud in 1895. Various states of consciousness, each characterized by styles of action and predominance of particular ideas and feelings, were described for the person exhibiting the hysterical phenomenon, an approach used in France by Charcot (1877) and Janet (1965). Breuer believed that the hypnoid state was of special etiological significance in the onset of symptoms. Indeed, a susceptibility to fluid state transition and multiple states of consciousness was thought to be a sign of a hysterical personality disorder.

The hysterical personality disorders (Horowitz, 1977a), as well as the narcissistic and borderline personality disorders (Kernberg, 1975; Kohut, 1977; Hartocollis, 1977), are characterized, in part, by the presence of distinctly different recurrent states. State distinctions can, however, be made for any person. For example, states vary from sleeping to waking, from high to low stress, from excitation to lethargy, from alertness to coma, from mood to mood, and from emotion to emotion. It is important, now, to extend state description beyond the context of severe personality disorders.

Any person's states and patterns of state transition are the behavioral manifestations of his character structure or personality. While flexibility in entering multiple states may be a sign of character strength, the inability to maintain a stable state may be a sign of character weakness. In persons with pathological or impaired character formation, states may seem more diverse and sharply delineated than those of persons with more mature levels of character development, where the transitions between states will be more modulated, subtle, and overlapping.

States common to most persons include those moments dominated by strong expression of emotions, such as anxiety, anger, guilt, sadness, shame, sexual excitement, surprise, and joy. However, each person experiences these general emotions in his own particular way. Each person may cry—the tissue box is a common fixture in the psychotherapist's office—but each person has his unique way of crying, emitting sounds, contorting facial muscles, experiencing sadness, and so forth. Enormous work has been done on the general aspects of emotion; little has been done to describe unique variations on such universal themes.

The most spectacular state transitions and state variations are noted in persons with multiple personalities and other types of dissociative phenomena. Sudden episodes of strong emotions are also clear shifts in state. Somewhat more subtle state variations require description of introspective experience. Federn (1952) studied a variety of states that he felt could not be categorized as dissociative episodes or as episodes of specific emotions and called them "ego states." He found evidence that the ego states of earlier developmental periods remained throughout life as potentially recurrent in behavior and experience. These might emerge during pathological or normal regressions. For example, the phenomenon can be elicited clearly by hypnotic age regression in normal persons (Weiss, 1960). Psychiatrist Eric Berne (1961, 1964) was a theoretician who built upon Federn's work. He founded a school of therapy out of general theory of ego states and called it transactional analysis. He classified the overall states of persons as adult, child, and parent. It was his thesis that each person had within himself these three characteristic roles for existing in the world and experiencing himself and others. In any two-person system, such as a marriage or a love affair, there were six personifications in action; each party could be in a child, parent, or adult state. By examining these states and state transitions, various repetitive transactions could be defined as pastimes, games, or true mutuality.

This simplification allowed a transactional analysis of recurrent patterns that led to changes in state. For example, an adult-to-adult interchange between husband and wife might shift when one party took on a parental role and addressed the other as if he were a child, perhaps through some form of criticism. One type of state would be ensured if the respondent accepted and enacted a dependent role. But another state, one of vindictive hostility, might ensue if the respondent also entered a parental ego state and counterattacked as if the spouse were a child.

Transactional analysis leads to description of the games people play and the states the games lead them through, but it tends to skim past description of the states that people seldom allow themselves to experience or experience but do not communicate in behavior. They dread such states enough to work at avoiding their recognition. These states are sometimes defended against by the development and perpetuation of the repeated behavior patterns described by Berne. Depth psychology requires acknowledgment and description of these warded-off states. It also requires the recognition of ideal states, which the transactional analysis system tends to omit. While these are seldom manifest, they are of motivational importance.

Continued work in the phenomenology of clinical psychology also indicated the necessity for describing a multiplicity of recurrent states for a given person. Bibring (1953) described the multiple states of the depressed person, and Kernberg (1975) is prominent among those who have shown the importance of describing different ego states for borderline and narcissistic characters. Kernberg (1975) and Mayman (1968) have proposed to differentiate these multiple states according to the object relationships that typified each period.

METHOD OF STATE DESCRIPTION

As information is reviewed, a first provisional list of states and descriptions is revised and fleshed out. The form and content of characteristic subjective experiences and of behavior are included. Seldom-experienced states can be added to fill out the picture.

It often helps to begin by describing the state of mind that contains the symptom, problem, or phenomenon of main interest in Step 1. This may immediately place several state descriptions onto a provisional list, if there are several phemonena of interest and they occur in different states of mind. When symptoms are the key phenomena, the states containing them are often experienced, or look to others, as being under-modulated. That is, the person seems to be having experiences and expressing behavior in a manner that is not well controlled in the sense of being under volitional management.

From that point, one can go on to list other undermodulated states, proceeding to well-modulated states. A list of states can indeed often usefully be divided into three categories: undermodulated, relatively well modulated, and overmodulated. Overmodulated states are those that seem to have rigid control features, sometimes leading to a sense of contrivance or pretense as well as restraint over expressions and experiences.

Such a listing of overcontrolled, well-modulated, and undercontrolled states has within it, even at this superficial level of formulation, the idea of conflict between impulses and regulatory, perhaps defensive, efforts. Once a series of states of mind are relatively well understood, this may lead to a reorganization of states into categories, such as those states that are desired by the person, those states the person dreads to enter, and those states that are compromises between such wishes and fears. This presents a provisional motivational view of the individual that can be enhanced by including states the individual considers as sought-after ideal ones, even though he or she may currently be unable to achieve them.

Once such lists of states and ideas about their motivational arrangements have been set forth, it is possible to use the state labels to discuss the nature of occurrence of each more important state. The triggers or events that influence the subject to enter the given state may be described. These may include social, psychological, and biological events, such as a change in situation, an emergent dream, the effect of drugs, or growing fatigue, as well as a life event of some magnitude. A model of state transitions that occur frequently can lead to a state cycle description. The nature of state transitions, whether abruptly explosive, smooth, or somewhere in between may also be an important feature worthy of careful description.

Illustration

Janice complained of depressions. In the problem list these were characterized as behavioral signs of apathy, withdrawal with feelings of fogginess and unreality, and overeating. This readily lends itself to a state description. From the data of the entire therapy, a label was selected for this state that seemed more informative, and more individualized than "depressed mood." This label was *hurt and not working*, a description that she used. She could recognize herself as entering and leaving this state. When it occurred, she felt dull and lonely, had bodily concerns, and tended to withdraw from social contacts and life tasks. When she entered this state during the treatment situation, she could be observed to mumble and trail off.

Other states were commonly observed but did not overlap as much with items from the problem list. One of her most frequent states was dramatic animation, when she felt as if she were pretending for the benefit of another person. In another frequent state she continued her efforts to work but felt and appeared as if her feelings were hurt. This was labeled the *hurt but working* state. Using her own words for the animated episodes, this was called the *tra-la-la* state. From such beginnings a list of states is formed, focusing on her inner experiences, as reported, and her manifest behavior, as observed (see Table 4).

Table 4. List of States

1. *Tra-la-la*	She is cheerful, lighthearted, entertaining, pretending
2. *Hurt but working*	She seems deflated but goes on with her tasks
3. *Hurt and not working*	She appears insulated or aloof, stops tasks, withdraws from contact with others
4. *Crying*	Unrestrained, open weeping. Displays weeping to others to solicit attention
5. *Competitive*	She ranges from a covert struggle for one-up position, to open anger with others, to placing blame upon others
6. *Acute self-disgust*	She is dismayed about some self-realization, with sensation of deflation

A more detailed state description included recurrent ideational themes, actions, and sensations. The aim was to base these descriptions on communications and observation, not on inference. For example, where the table says "crying-weeping with display to others to elicit attention," it means that **she described herself as crying to elicit attention**; this was not an inference by the observer about what her crying **might** mean.

An example of the closeness of state description to direct material can be seen in the following excerpts from transcripts of the therapy. During the second therapy session she had been describing her irritation with her low status at work and how, even in such an undemanding role, her efforts were criticized as inadequate. The therapist commented that she felt degraded at work and then asked if that concept also applied to the therapy situation. This was part of his effort to understand why a working alliance was slow in development. As will be seen, she responded by switching between affirmation and denial (a habitual style to be discussed in a subsequent step). She did work with the concept, however, and gradually referred to her use of the *tra-la-la* state to avoid states of feeling and seeming *hurt*. While describing how she airily told friends she was in therapy, her manner was buoyant and lighthearted. This state prevented her from feeling bad when admitting she needed therapy.

Excerpt from Second Hour of Therapy

T: So, with this kind of idea you're vulnerable to feeling kind of degraded.

P: MmHm [long pause].

T: Well, how about, how about being a patient here? Does that have any current of being degraded?

P: MmHm [pause]. It does and it doesn't. I mean I've been a lot happier since, since making the decision of actually coming here.

T: MmHm.

P: And, like all this past week I went around feeling happy and feeling good. And, you know, a little stronger and stuff. And I knew that it was because I had done something that I hope will be good for me. But at the same time I, yeah, I don't go around telling everybody. Like I'm not going to tell my family, to them that [therapy] would be degrading. What's wrong with you, you shouldn't talk to outsiders. You shouldn't. Oh, you're so weird, you're always so weird [pause]. And, uh, I make a joke out of it when I tell my friends. "Guess what! Tra-la-tra-la and for free! Tra-la-la-la and I'm on tape!" That aspect of it, you know, nothing about why and . . . [said lightheartedly, but she trails off and falls silent].

T: Yeah, well, that sounds a little like you're **telling them** not to take it seriously.

P: MmHm.

T: It's just a lark.

P: MmHm. I'm not allowed to take it seriously.

T: **Yeah**.

P: Why am I here? In fact I almost didn't come today [said more seriously]. I'm, I don't need to come here.

T: Well, you're afraid to take it seriously.

P: Yeah. And, yeah, and all I can say, you know, like I **can't** say there's something wrong with me. I can't, well, for one thing that's, you know, that's the always too dramatic, right? If I sat down and I said, I'm really worried and I'm really unhappy, and, uh, part of me would say [whispers], "O, wow, there she goes again. She loves being center stage."

T: Uh, huh.

P: And so I have to say, Well, it's 'cause I'm tired of being depressed. And I know there's some things I want to change and I know I can't do it myself. So this is one way of doing it. And that's what I say, if anything, to my friends. I think that's what I said to Phillip. You know he was really concerned. I just kind of popped in and said, "Oh, guess what I'm going to start doing." And he said, "Eh," and he kind of came back a few minutes later and he was really concerned, "Why are you doing this?"

T: Mm.

P: "I didn't know you were unhappy," he didn't say that but, you know.

T: Yeah, **he** took it seriously.

P: MmHm. And so I told him, well, you know, I've been depressed. You remember this, you remember that. And I can't do it by myself. So I'm going to do it. And he accepted that [pause]. And, and, I mean, I wasn't going to tell him [pause] anything else [pause]. See, I'm not even going to say it **now** [laugh] [pause].

T: Well, I'm not going to force you to either.

P: Yeah. Well, see, I still feel like I'm, **I'm being dramatic**. What is she keeping under cover? What can't she even admit to herself? [Dramatically and archly said] Tune in next week.

T: That might be right.

P: [Laughs] That just goes with the feeling of unreality. I can't even evaluate myself.

T: Yeah. Well, look, you've been checking up on both of us and this situation. And it's a style of yours, you know. A style of yours is to be very private and secret, I think.

P: You know, one of the tools I use to do that is to act very, very open.

T: Mm.

P: I'm more open than anybody I know as far as what I'll say about myself, and, and [pause].

T: Yeah, yeah.

P: And I go around embarrassing people because I tell their secrets, too.

T: Yeah.

P: I've known that, I've just never said it.

Excerpt from Third Hour of Therapy

Other examples of both the *hurt but working* and the *tra-la-la* states are found in the next session, the third therapy interview. For the first time she described the funeral for her brother as a kind of reevaluation of the relationship between herself and her parents. Material from the later phase of therapy indicated that this theme was extremely important. But at this early point in therapy she was warding off recognition of its implications. In the excerpt that follows she gradually entered the dramatic *tra-la-la* state as she imitated her parents' comments about how weird she was. Although this shift in state is most dramatic and clear on videotape where the nonverbal behavior emphasizes the meanings, it is also conveyed in language as transcribed.

T: So the trip back for the funeral was also a kind of reevaluation for you and your parents.

P: MmHm.

T: Where they sat you down and had these talks with you.

P: Yeah, and indicated that although they didn't like it [her relationship with Phillip], they had suddenly discovered that they were prejudiced, that they minded very much, they were worried about our rel—, what our relatives would say, they were worried about me, and, you know, potential problems, and all that. I was kind of hurt at some of the stuff they brought up because it sounded like they didn't think I had thought much about it. But, of course, by their view of some of the things I've done, I never think at all. I do all these amazingly stupid things [sniff].

T: So, according to their version, I mean, we both know we're caricaturing it a little bit, you're kind of a nymphomaniac, just running all over . . .

P: [interrupts] "I'm weird, weird . . . " (dramatic and lighthearted).
T: San Francisco and sleeping with everybody.
P: Mm, ahh, Daddy told me I was, I always had been kind of kinky or some-
    thing like that.

As she continued on this line, she became progressively dramatic and entered more into the pretending *tra-la-la* state. She used her words for this state in the following excerpt, where the therapist persisted in trying to get at her own feelings about herself.

P: [Loud voice] Also because I like the idea of the atmosphere and **trala-trala-trala** . . . With them it's a commie-hippie-weirdo college and the only reason I want to go there is because I'm still rebelling. And, and on, and on, and just [pause].
T: I guess you feel undermined.
P: [Whispers really softly] Undermined? [Normal volume] I don't know, I had, I mean I had to get away from them [her parents], I can't deal with something when it's real close. One thing that makes it really hard is that we are very close. I mean, we're a tight-knit family and I, I really love them [cough]. And so it's, you know, it's not as if I can just push them off and say, ah, whatever [sniff].

Inclusion of Seldom Experienced Warded-Off and Ideal States

Because states are experiential they can be remembered or fantasied as well as expressed. Past states as well as possible future states are contemplated, and the desire for or fear of such states can be an influential source of motivation. That is why a list of states can include those that occur rarely but have important status in terms of wishes and threats.

For example, the state of *acute self-disgust* was included in the sample list. Janice seldom entered this state, and exited from it rapidly. While rarely experienced, it was a major threat for her, a state warded off in a variety of ways because it was extremely painful to experience. A desired or ideal state may also be added to the list. How was she trying to feel when, by her own volition, she was in the *tra-la-la* state? From what she said in therapy, she wished to feel competent, engaged with another, self-confident, happy, frank, honest, and womanly. This would be an ideal state, one of *authentic working*, the achievement of which was an important goal, and motivation for her behavior.

Details are added that may include the form and content of verbal and nonverbal communications observed during therapy. With elaboration of details one may obtain a fuller description of states, as illustrated in Table 5, according to an under-, well-, and overmodulated format.

Information derived at any time can be used to describe the states for the early period, before change has taken place. This is important because sometimes change is necessary before the person can express or even become aware of some aspects of his previous behavior.

Closeness to Observation

Note that descriptions in Table 5 apply to behavior and conscious experiences. But even at the level of state description there is great abstraction, simplification, classification, and use of low-level clinical inference to arrive at judgments. Multiple layers of experience are common. Since states are experiential, they can be modeled in the mind and used as memories or fantasies, as past or future as well as present expressions. They can be durable or momentary, semisimultaneous or independent. Janice would, for example, attempt to enter one state while at the same time she was in danger of experiencing another state. She would try to enter the *tra-la-la* state when she was vulnerable to feeling *self-disgusted* or *hurt*. She would try to display this vivacity, but her face might suddenly and quite briefly lose its composure and show a troubled expression. Such acts of will to change or maintain states are common efforts toward self-control. There may also be split manifestations, a *tra-la-la* state expressed in speech with a *hurt* state indicated by facial expression and other bodily signals.

Transitions between States

Once states are recognizable, one can ask when they are entered and when they change to another state. This step also requires low-level clinical inference but is anchored as close to observation as possible by a focus on external events rather than inner motivations. Inner reasons are examined later. Here, one states the patterns of communication, interpersonal behavior, and the life events or environmental shifts that are repeatedly associated with a change in states. As with listing the states, one begins with tentative, diffuse, even vague statements and then sharpens them by repeated observation.

Illustration. For example, Janice frequently shifted from the *tra-la-la* state to the *hurt but working* state. This shift occurred early in therapy, whenever the therapist actively confronted her with concepts she wished to avoid. If she came too close to expressing these warded-off contents she was in danger of entering a state of *acute self-disgust*. On the other hand, whenever she could cope well or successfully institute a defensive

Table 5. Description of Recurrent States by Degree of Modulation

Label	Description
Undermodulated states	
Acute self-disgust, shame, or despair (dreaded)	Feels revulsion at being fat, unaccomplished; self-critical, inactive, withdrawn, silly, pretending, or sexually wrong (too active, too inactive). Most other states are to ward off this one.
Hurt and not working	Withdraws, reads, overeats, refuses social invitations, mumbles and trails off during interview; feels foggy and unreal; depressed, has bodily concerns, sad, lonely.
Well-modulated states	
Crying	Displays weeping to others to elicit attention.
Hurt but working	Head down, shamed or depressed; holding, rubbing, or picking self with hands, more leaden face, talks more slowly and softly; reflective on self, attention inward.
Authentic working (ideal state)	Competent, authentic, engaged, self-confident, happy, honest, womanly.
Competitive	Critical of or struggling with others to see who will control or dominate the situation, who is to blame if it doesn't go well; edge in voice, feels contempt, indignation, or anger; challenges other to prove worth; can escalate to temper outburst.
Overmodulated state	
Tra-la-la	Engaging, perky, histrionic; gestures are wide and outward, attention on other, smiles, makes faces, fast-talking, interrupts. Pretends to feel but is distant from the stated ideas. May play-act or exaggerate her own ideas and feelings while feeling inwardly at a distance from them. Would like to feel mutually engaged with another, or actively creative, but feels inwardly at a distance from these ideals as well.

maneuver after these confrontations, she would exit from the *hurt but working* state and return to the *tra-la-la* state.

Another transition occurred whenever she was abandoned by a person to whom she was attached, and had no replacement for this relationship. She would then change from her *tra-la-la* state to the *hurt and not working* state. Injury to self-esteem could also lead to the *hurt and not working* state but usually led first to a brief period of *acute self-disgust*. From the *hurt and not working* state she might enter the *crying* state if there was someone else present (see Figure 4). In another pattern relatively easy to observe when she felt *acute self-disgust*, she would quickly enter a *competitive* state if her interpersonal situation allowed her to blame someone else for shortcomings that were "in the air."

As indicated earlier, the two most frequent states Janice experienced were *tra-la-la* and *hurt but working*. An example of each has been given; a further episode from the first treatment hour illustrates her transition between states.

As part of his exploratory aims, the therapist was about to follow up on a piece of information Janice gave in passing, about living with a male partner. Her first response to his question was within her *tra-la-la* state, as seen by review of videotape and reflected in the transcript by her words, "Great! Fantastic!" The therapist then made Janice's statement more definite by repeating it firmly. In her response, she indicated a problem she wished to avoid, and then entered the *hurt but working* state, reflected in the transcript by speech disruptions and on videotape by a lowered vocal tone and facial expression. By the end of the brief excerpt cited below, she said, "I think that's just a prejudice." She left the *hurt but working* state and was once again in the *tra-la-la* state. The use of intellectualization as a defense helped her to make this transition.

T: Well, you say you have an old man. How are things going?
P: Great! Fantastic!
T: That's not blocked then.
P: [Sigh] [entry into *hurt but working* state] There's something there, that [pause] that I don't want to think about.
T: Mm.
P: Um [pause]. Like I, I, one of the reasons I'm afraid of, c-coming here, is I'm afraid that if it helps me get started thinking and growing and kind of heading toward being the person I want to be [pause] I'm afraid it'll mean I have to leave him.
T: MmHm.
P: But I don't know I, [entry into *tra-la-la* state] I also think that's just a prejudice I have, and that if I'm not miserable for somebody, or striving to be something I'm not or, you know.

State Cycles

From such observations it is possible to construct a larger scale model of the cycle of states. Such models have explanatory power; they demonstrate that if the patient is in a given state, and "something" happens to him, he will then enter another state.

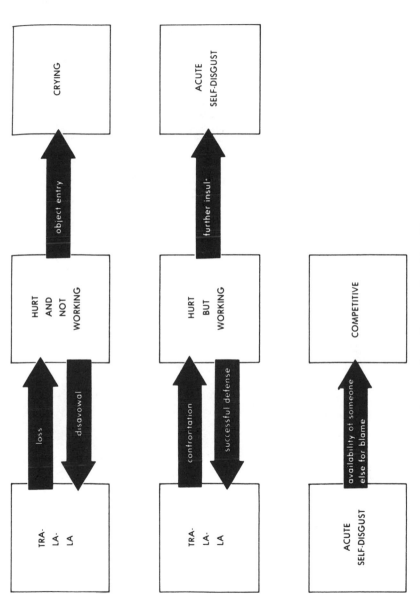

Figure 4. Some Common State Transitions.

    In constructing a cyclic model of states one can also include the
states that rarely occur.
    A cycle of states for Janice is shown in Figure 5. The most dreaded
state has already been described, that of *acute self-disgust*. The *ideal* state,
feeling authentically like an active competent woman in a state of mutuality with another person, seldom if ever occurred. The closest she could
usually manage to come was the *tra-la-la* state. She shifted to the *hurt
but working* state when reminded of her shortcomings or conflicts. With
successful defense against these threats to her self-esteem, she moved
back into the *tra-la-la* state (see Figure 5).

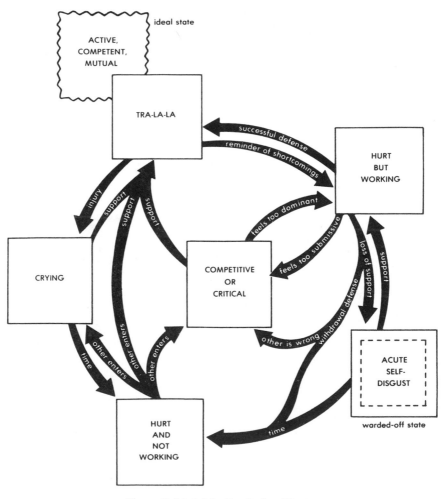

Figure 5. Model for the Cycle of States.

Excessive confrontation with her shortcomings in the absence of support from others led to her entry into the *acute self-disgust* state. She would not remain in that state for long; it was too painful. Instead, as shown in Figure 5, she attempted to avoid that state in one of two ways: She would either withdraw immediately and enter the *hurt and not working* state, or when someone else was available, enter the *competitive* state, and argue that this person was at fault. This had another advantage; through competition and challenge she engaged attention. If she gained sufficient support, as in intellectual argument, she could reenter the *tra-la-la* state. Another exit from the *competitive* state occurred when she felt too dominant. She then reentered the *hurt but working* state and felt less powerful. Conversely, when she felt too submissive she tended to shift from the *hurt but working* state to the *competitive* state.

Following Figure 5 clockwise, one notes that when there was both a blow to her self-esteem and an absence of support, she entered the *hurt and not working* state. The alternative was the state of *acute self-disgust*. This was rarely entered; when it was, she quickly changed into the less painful, more stable *hurt and not working* state.

SUMMARY

A list of recurrent states helps define an individual personality at a particular moment in his life history. This definition depends on observation of behavior and clear understanding of reported inner experiences. Naturally, empathy and open encounter can heighten state description. Since each person has many states, only the most relevant are abstracted. The given context defines what is relevant for each person, at a particular time, for a specific purpose.

For the purpose of change in maladaptive or painful states, problem states offer the point of departure. In this way, state description moves from particular presenting complaints toward problem states as they are embedded in an overall matrix of personal patterns.

While it focuses on the individual, state description can advance theories of psychopathology as typologies are examined for similarities and differences. For example, several persons with a given type of personality disorder can be studied to see what states are common to them and differ from those in groups of persons with another personality disorder. State description will also help observation of patterns of change. Furthermore, labeling of states can help both patient and therapist by heightening awareness of reasons for entry into problem states and state transition patterns.

Table 6. Dictionary of States of Mind[a]

Affective Sets

1. Sadness	5. Tension	9. Affection
2. Fear/anxiety	6. Dullness	10. Creative excitement
3. Self-disgust/shame/guilt	7. Communication	11. Joy
4. Anger	8. Engagement	12. Sexual excitement

Undermodulated	Modulated	Overmodulated
1. Sadness		
Distraught sadness	Quietly needy	As if sad
Out-of-control crying	Crying	Phony poignancy
Demoralized and deflated	Struggle against crying	As if remorseful
Desperately overwhelmed	Poignantly empathic	
	Unhappily vulnerable	
2. Fear/anxiety		
Bodily panic	Fearful worry	As if anxious
Panicky emptiness	Apprehensive vigilance	Numbing from fear
Frightened vulnerability	Mixed shame/rage/fear	
Panicky helplessness	Nervously irritable	
3. Self-disgust/shame/guilt		
Shameful mortification	Shamed, disgrace, bashful shyness, remorseful, self-disgust, angry self-disgust	As if self-disgusted or guilty
	Remorse	
	Whining	
Revolted self-disgust	Hurt attentiveness	
Intrusive guilt	Mixed shame/rage/fear	
Panicky guilt		
4. Anger		
Explosive fury	Angry	As if angry
Panicky rage	Bitter	Blustering
Self-righteous rage	Resentful	Cutely angry
Grandiose bellicosity	Annoyed, skeptical	
Tantrum	Sniping	
	Whining	
Defiance		
Shame/rage/fear		
5. Tension		
Excitedly disorganized	Tentative engagement	As if strained
Confused	Struggle with vulnerability	
Overwhelmed and pained		
Hypervigilant		
Anxious and withdrawn		
Distracted		

Table 6. (*Continued*)

Undermodulated	Modulated	Overmodulated
6. Dullness		
Foggy withdrawal	Bored	Coldly remote
Listless apathy	Meandering	
Fugue or coma		
Hurt and unengaged		
7. Communication		
Pressured confusion	Assured, productive, compassionate	Rigid reporting
Pressured dumping	Composed, authentic	Technical display
Frenzied activity	Earnest activity	As if bold
		Pontification
		Controlled documentarian
8. Engagement		
Giddy engagement	Composed, authentic	As if bold
Foolishly excited, histrionic	Earnest activity	Pontification
	Elated and poised	Social chitchat
	Shining (smiling, beaming)	Snide sociability
		As if light hearted
9. Affection		
Foolishly enthralled	Tenderness	Coyly ingratiating
Overawed	Assured compassion	As if light-hearted
10. Creative excitement		
Excited hyperactivity	Oceanic	As if illuminated
Frenzied creativity or "good" activity	Illuminated	
Shining (smiling, beaming)	Creative flow	
11. Joy		
Foolishly enthralled	Cheerful	As if light hearted
Foolishly excited, histrionic	Sharing	Social chitchat
		Coyly ingratiating
12. Sexual excitement		
Enthralled love	Flirtatious pleasure	As if eroticized
Flooded with eroticism	Eroticized sensuality	
Sexual titillated		

*Sometimes a label for a state of mind is on "the tip of the tongue" but is hard to phrase. These are some terms that may help in labeling states of mind. They are arranged in emotion and degree of modulation. The 12 emotional colorations are listed first, then with under-, well-, and overmodulated state names.

CHAPTER THREE

Self-Concepts and
Role Relationship Models

Step 3. Interpersonal Behavioral Patterns, Self-Concepts, and Role Relationship Models: *Describe the recurrent maladaptive interpersonal behavioral patterns that are related to the problems as defined in Steps 1 and 2. Then infer and describe the intrapsychic person schemata, motives, and personal agendas upon which these maladaptive patterns are based. When there is sufficient information, reconstruct the probable development of the views contained in these schemata.*

A. Repertoire of Self- and Object Schemata: *List the self- and object concepts of the person, and describe his or her highest development achievement in terms of integrating these into supraordinate views.*

B. Role Relationship Models: *Organize the self- and object views into models that suggest complementarity in aims and expectations of response. Relate each state in Step 2 to these role relationship models, attempting to posit the main model for a given state.*

C. Scripts, Schematic Agendas, and Story Lines: *Describe schematic sequences of role relationship models as they are inferred to underlie repetitive maladaptive interpersonal patterns.*

D. Relationship Conflicts: *Model conflicts and/or deficiencies surrounding the personal agenda of the individual at the present life developmental period. Include regressive as well as progressive aims. Describe how recent life events may have activated latent conflictual relationship themes or warded off self-concepts.*

In the previous step, multiple states of mind for the individual were described. Part of the description focused on subjective experiences of self and other, and the style of interpersonal transaction that characterized each state. This step goes from those observations and subjective self-reports to inferences about the schematic structures of meanings that lead to similar patterns when a given state recurs. The assumption is made that each state of mind tends to use as organizers certain schemata from a larger available repertoire of the individual. The most important schemata under consideration are those that may be called *person schemata* because they organize wholistic views of the self or another person.

In addition to person schemata, other schemata include scripts of sequences of interactions that might take place, and templates for how to form interpersonal action plans. Schemata tend to endure once they have developed, but new variants can form as the consequence of recognizing new experiences and learning from them (Bartlett, 1932; Piaget, 1937/1954; see also Kagan, 1982; Stern, 1984).

While the object relations view has permeated psychodynamics and the concept of self has long been a part of social learning theory and developmental psychology, one aspect of the theory used as the basis of configurational analysis is not so familiar. This is the idea that an individual has multiple self-concepts. Of course, the idea of polypsychism does go back to the eras of Mesmerism and hypnosis and is contained in the ideas of Jung, Freud, and Janet, as summarized by Ellenberger (1964). Yet seeing the individual *both* as a singular self-organization *and* as having multiple self-concepts is not generally accepted. It is possible to have one's cake and eat it too on this issue by viewing self-schematic issues as a nested hierarchy that does not always result in a unitary self-organization that matches the unity of the physical body. The issue of multiple self-schemata, and even multiple "brains" in one person, the right and left hemispheres, if disconnected (Sperry, 1966), can be addressed. The issue of "who decides" on intrapsychic intentions can also be addressed. To do so, some definitions of terms to expand on the word *self* are necessary. These are terms as they will be used throughout the rest of this text.

DEFINITIONS

1. *Self* will be used in the commonplace manner to mean overall personal reference.
2. *Self-concept* will be used to describe a view that has at least once been conscious and is a part of knowledge that can again be

consciously represented for self-reflective thought and communication.

3. *Self-schema* will be used to describe an organization of information into a unit which pertains—rightly or wrongly—to the self but which is not necessarily conscious or capable of access to conscious or communicative representation. Nonetheless, self-schemata may function unconsciously to help organize thought and action.

4. *Supraordinate* self-concepts or schemata are higher-order forms that contain, in a nested and integrated way, several self-concepts or schemata. A *supraordinate self-concept* would allow a person to consciously reflect upon himself as composed of more than one personality configuration, and so as having different experiences about a theme in varied states of mind. A *supraordinate self-schemata* would make possible unconscious integrations across changing motives and perceived circumstances.

5. A *role relationship model* contains views of self as related to others. These could be concepts or schemata or both. In a role relationship model of the association between the self and one other person there will be at least four components:
   a. The characteristics and role of the self.
   b. The characteristics and role of the other.
   c. The motives, intentions, expectations, and defenses that lead to aims of self toward the other.
   d. The view of the aims, expectations, and likely responses of the other toward the self.

6. Sequences of role relationship models may be schematized as well into units called *scripts, scenarios,* or *story lines*. When such sequences gain intentional status and are stored as purposes, they could be called *agendas*. Such schemata act as plans for action sequences and may be released into active function as organizers of information when trigger situations occur.

BACKGROUND

A self-schemata and role relationship model may be activated when such schemata are associated with the possibility of gratifying a wish or coping with a fear. Freud, in his exploration of the Oedipus complex as a "family romance," exposed the unconscious persistence and dynamic power of early interpersonal relationship patterns throughout adult life (Freud, 1905/1953b, 1909/1959a, 1912/1955a, 1912/1958a). Jung's theory of the archetypes contained the idea of multiple, unconscious self-schemata (Stevens, 1982). Rapaport (1967) and Knapp (1969) later elaborated upon the preconscious, conscious, and unconscious layers of such relationship fantasies.

Arlow (1969) also explored the importance to decision making and behavior of relatively enduring and stable fantasies of specific self-concepts, views of others, and story lines as developed unconsciously and persisting unconsciously. These motivationally infused schemata include role relationship models and scripts of both pleasurable and traumatic transactions. In order to prevent the unconsciously anticipated threatening aspects of these agenda, controls are instituted that may prevent conscious concepts. Anna Freud (1936) continued Sigmund Freud's work in clarifying how defense mechanisms warded off not only specific memories and fantasies but self- and object concepts as well, as she defined role reversal, identification with the aggressor, and altruistic surrender to identification with the goals of another person.

Federn (1952) described how different states of behavior were associated with different self-feelings, findings elaborated by Schilder (1950) and Sullivan (1953). Berne (1961) explained different ego states by different self-concepts as child, parent, or adult. What Arlow and Knapp refer to as central interpersonal fantasies Berne saw as the variety of possible interactions between such self- and other concepts. Berne recognized the two major limitations of his method. There were, for example, many more possible roles than child, adult, and parent. He attempted to solve this problem by subdividing each role, as in the example of a child subrole as "the Little Professor." Unfortunately, his method of transactional analysis was encumbered by the use of only a few general categories.

More categories have been provided by the interpersonal circle method for scoring recurrent, complementary interpersonal patterns. These include axes for kindness to hostility, domination to subordination, and autonomy to dependence (Benjamin, 1979; Wiggins, 1979, 1982; Kiesler, 1983). These could be used in configurational analysis, but here a wider range of individualized description will be advocated.

My own work, in the first edition of this book, followed the clarification of self-representation as being multiple in individuals that is found in the work of Hartmann (1950/1977), Sullivan (1953), Erikson (1954), Jacobson (1964), Kohut (1971, 1977), and Kernberg (1975), as well as in the writings of the British Object Relations School (from M. Klein, 1948, to Bowlby, 1969, 1973, 1980), and work on moral development, which is well summarized by Loevinger (1976). I attempted to clarify by careful case-by-case analysis the operation of multiple self-concepts, schemata, and role relationship models in different states of mind and as consciously and unconsciously operative (Horowitz, 1977a). I analyzed state transitions as explosive or smooth, as regressive or progressive, in terms of the degree to which these different forms were coherent in larger-order, supraordinate structures (Horowitz, 1979; Horowitz and Zilberg, 1983).

Working from a different tradition, that of personality trait psychology, Kelly (1955) developed a system based on defining the core constructs a person habitually uses in appraisals of himself and others. This led to considerable research on how interpersonal views are organized, and indicated a fair degree of consciousness even about usually warded-off views (Bannister, 1985; Neimeyer, 1986).

Person schemata terms, as used in cognitive psychology, are in essence the same as defined here (see Singer and Salovey, in press, for a review). The sequential schemata operating unconsciously when motivated are called core operating principles by Meichenbaum and Gilmore (1984). Markus (1977; Markus and Smith, 1981) has demonstrated variance in how persons differ as to the way they handle information depending on their schemata for a given kind of trait. Fiske and Taylor (1984), Schank and Abelson (1977), Berne (1964), Tomkins (1979), Bower, Black, and Turner (1979), and Carlson and Carlson (1984) have provided work on how scripts operate out of awareness as organizing forms in social information processing. The psychodynamic point of view adds motives, conflict between motives, and defensive regulation to these theories.

These advances suggest that methods that summarize person schemata can explain important intrusions and omissions in patterns of interpersonal transaction. Intrusions are misapplications of inner views due to strong motives to impose these role relationship models. Omissions are states in which the realistic properties of interpersonal situations seem to be ignored in favor of personal stereotypes that are projected onto the situation.

METHOD

Included in Janice's list of complaints (Table 3, Chapter One, p. 23) were those made during therapy about her inability to motivate herself to work, and her recognition of a recurrent maladaptive interpersonal relationship pattern of being too passive-aggressive, dependent, dramatic, or pretending with others. Furthermore, the therapist described, as problems he formulated, Janice's inferred defective self-concepts and an unresolved ambivalent attachment to her mother. He said her aims for independence and dependence acting in conflict led to interpersonal struggles over who would be in control. These interpersonal behavioral patterns and recurrent self-concepts can now be described in a series of substeps subdivided into (a) repertoire of self- and object schemata, (b) role relationship models, (c) scripts, agendas, and story lines, and (d) relationship conflicts.

Repertoire of Self- and Object Schemata

In this substep we will list Janice's self- and object concepts and then make an inference about her level of developing supraordinate schematic forms.

Repertoire of Self-Concepts. Self-concepts for each state of mind may be listed by reviewing as many instances as possible of the specific state of mind and inferring the self-view that is its major organizing principle. Each different state, as listed in Step 2, does not have to have a different self-concept in this assembly of the repertoire of self-schemata. States may vary according to the status of organizers other than self-schemata.

It is usually best to start with the most observable recurrent states. A result for Janice is shown in Table 7.

Repertoire of Object Concepts. One can also list major object concepts or schemata that seem to serve as predominant organizers in each state of mind. Since roles are readily taken as self or other, some of the same

Table 7. Relationship of Janice's States to Her Self-Concepts

State	Recurrent self-concepts
Tra-la-la	"As if" an active, competent, creative, and sexual woman, sometimes as if an exceptionally gifted person
Hurt but working	Impaired but learning student
Hurt and not working	Alone, self-sufficient because nothing can be expected from others (warded-off yearning for others)
Crying	Weak, wounded waif; deserving of help, yearning for others
Competitive	Strong, wrongly criticized, inadequately provided for by others
Acute self-digust, shame, or *despair*	Defective, fat, lazy, immature, like mother (or "mother's girl") or also sexually wrong, greedy, nastily selfish
Ideal	Active, competent, sexual, creative

labels for object concepts may be used as in the list of self-concepts. For example, Janice was concerned that she might be too dependent on having her mother as the global source of her identity, and this meant we could infer an object concept as "essential supplier of identity," as opposed to some other role that would be not overpowering but acceptable, as in viewing another person as a good teacher.

Janice also indicated that she feared others acting in a superior role and judging her critically. Sometimes she reversed the roles and viewed them as deserving scorn because they were defective or bad in their habits. The role of superior critic is thus an important one.

Organizational Level of Self- and Object Schematization. Next, one can draw inferences about the highest level the person has achieved in terms of nesting different self- and object schemata into more complex but integrated organizations. One can also state the current level of functioning. This may be different from the highest level of self-organization previously achieved if regression has occurred. It will be easier to progress to use of an already developed supraordinate schemata than to develop such a higher-order form for the first time. This has implications for treatment technique as well as prognosis.

Gedo and Goldberg (1973) suggested a useful classification for this purpose which was cast into a table in the first edition of this book (1979). Since then my colleagues and I have found that ratings on the levels of self- and object schematization, as shown here in Table 8, were associated with the process and outcome of therapy in just such cases as that of Janice (Horowitz, Marmar, Weiss, DeWitt, and Rosenbaum, 1984). In addition, work by Hartley, Geller, and Behrends (1985) has indicated the value of such efforts, although we are still at a rudimentary level of understanding the development of person schemata.

Gedo and Goldberg describe persons at the lowest of five levels of self-cohesiveness and role relationships, Mode 1, as those who, during the period under examination, are unable to differentiate self from other, and demonstrate thought and behavior that is a relatively reflexive response to stimulation or drives. The next lowest level, Mode 2, classifies persons who can differentiate self from other, but whose self- and other concepts contain massive distortions of information. The self-concepts of such persons are often grandiose, and their inner models of others are often idealized. These self- and other concepts are not wholes but are part self and part others, often regarded as self-extensions or self-objects (Kohut, 1977). A person with fragmentary self-concepts and delusionary beliefs about self and other would be classified in this mode.

Table 8. Judgment of Organizational Level of Self- and Object Schematization

Mode 5.	The person has a well-developed supraordinate self-schema and functions from a relatively unitary position about familiar concerns. He has conflicts, of course, but these are between various realistic choices and various interpersonal possibilities or limitations of real relationships. His internal character conflicts have been relatively well resolved, perhaps through the use of renunciations, sublimations, choices, wisdom, humor, or even resignation. The person is able to experience others as separate persons with equivalent characteristics to his own. That is, he sees others as experiencing inner feelings, needs, reactions, memories, and fantasies, just as he does.
Mode 4.	There is a solidly differentiated supraordinate self-schema. However, in some areas the person experiences contradictory aims within that supraordinate self-concept. For example, the person may see himself as both wanting to express some aim in behavior and opposing such expression on moral grounds. Both the aim and the injunction against behavior are experienced as self-owned. Neurotic conflicts about sexuality and power that are not externalized or split might indicate this mode of function.
Mode 3.	The person has an incomplete supraordinate self-schematization. He is able to maintain a cohesive and relatively realistic self-view, but there are limited areas of exception, vulnerability to a sense of loss of self-concept cohesion, or to externalization and internalization at an unrealistic level. For example, a person with omnipotent illusions confined to the sphere of sexuality would be assigned this mode, as would a person who consistently disowned particular aggressive behavior although it was flagrantly obvious to others.
Mode 2.	The person has reached self-differentiation from others but has not yet been able to stabilize self-cohesion that includes positive and negative traits. Rather, he has various independently organized self-schemata that are each only part of the actual self-organization and various concepts of others that include only part of the actual behavior of others. Some others may be viewed as self-extensions or self-objects. Persons with massively deteriorated self-concepts and concepts without recurrent recognition of deflections of such views from reality would fall into this mode.
Mode 1.	Self- and other differentiation is at best only partial; there is significant confusion of self with other, or self and other are regarded as intermixed.

To be classified at the middle level, or Mode 3, the person must be able to maintain a cohesive and relatively realistic self-concept. In relation to some conflicts, such as those between sexual aims and sexual restrictions, there may be split-off nonintegrated self-concepts and role relationship models. For example, a person with consistent delusions of his own omnipotence only in the sphere of sexuality might be classified as having advanced to this level if in other spheres he maintains relatively realistic views of self and other.

The fourth and fifth modes are characterized by integrity and cohesion of the self-concept. In Mode 4 there is conflict between disparate aims within the self. The person may, for example, be aware of strong sexual wishes that are opposed by strong personal taboos. In Mode 5, the highest level of functioning, conflicts between the self and others may occur in real interactions, although the internal model of the self is relatively unified and realistic in all spheres. Where conflict once existed, consistent decisions and renunciations have taken place and a unified position on most issues exists.

Janice has reached the stage of coherent self-representation, albeit with conflicts, and so would be classified in Mode 4, although she is not firmly entrenched at this level. The equivalent position for Janice on the Loevinger (1976, pp. 25–26) categorization of milestones of ego development (Table 9) would be that of the Individualistic Stage. That is, she respects individuality, is having an emotional problem with dependence, has achieved self-separation and recognition of others, and differentiates between her inner and external life. She is beyond the stages Loevinger defined as Conformity and Conscientious but has not achieved the stability of Autonomous or Integrated levels of development.

Role Relationship Models

The lists of concepts of self and others will provide a beginning from which to construct role relationship models. Each element entered suggests complementary roles facilitating pattern observations in repeated reviews of available information.

As already mentioned, a role relationship model includes at least four elements: a self-concept or role; the role of the other person; a desire, intention, or feeling toward the other; and an expected action or reaction from the other. These may include expressions of emotion, desires, or wishful appetites, as well as threat expectations. A three-person role relationship model would include additional features, like a view such as envy for the bond between the two others.

Terms for roles can be selected using combinations of such nouns and adjectives as shown in the open-ended dictionary of Table 10; terms for expected or intended actions can be selected from such lists of aims, intentions, and expectations as are shown in Table 11.

Once again, it is helpful to begin with the most salient or repeated states of mind. For Janice the most frequent states were *tra-la-la* and *hurt but working*. The danger of entering a painful state of *acute self-disgust* was motivationally important to the oscillation between these states. One may add role relationships to a model of these transitions. An

Table 9. Some Milestones of Self-Development[a]

Stage	Code	Impulse control character development	Interpersonal style	Conscious preoccupations	Cognitive style
Presocial	I-1		Autistic	Self versus nonself	
Symbiotic impulsive	I-2	Impulsive, fear of retaliation	Symbiotic Receiving, dependent, exploitative	Bodily feelings, especially sexual and aggressive	Stereotyping, conceptual confusion
Self-protective	Δ	Fear of being caught, externalizing blame, opportunistic	Wary, manipulative, exploitative	Self-protection, trouble, wishes, things, advantage, control	
Conformist	I-3	Conformity to external rules, shame, guilt for breaking rules	Belonging, superficial niceness	Appearance, social acceptability, banal feelings, behavior	Conceptual simplicity, stereotypes, cliches
Conscientious-conformist	I-3/4	Differentiation of norms, goals	Aware of self in relation to group, helping	Adjustment, problems, reasons, opportunities (vague)	Multiplicity
Conscientious	I-4	Self-evaluated standards, guilt for consequences, long-term goals and ideals	Intensive, responsible, mutual, concern for communication	Differentiated feelings, motives for behavior, self-respect, achievements, traits, expression	Conceptual complexity, idea of patterning
Individualistic	I-4/5	Add:[b] Respect for individuality	Add: Dependence as an emotional problem	Add: Development, social problems, differentiation of inner life from outer	Add: Distinction of process and outcome
Autonomous	I-5	Add: Coping with conflicting inner needs, toleration	Add: Respect for autonomy, interdependence	Vividly conveyed feelings, integration of physiological and psychological causation of behavior, role conception, self-fulfillment, self in social context	Increased conceptual complexity, complex patterns, toleration for ambiguity, broad scope objectivity
Integrated	I-6	Add: Reconciling inner conflicts, renunciation of unattainable	Add: Cherishing of individuality	Add: Identity	

[a]From Loevinger, 1976, pp. 25–26, where it is called Ego Development.
[b]Add means in addition to the description applying to the previous level.

Table 10. A Dictionary of Terms for Labeling Self- and Object Concepts in Role Relationship Models

Some nouns

Companion	Exploiter	Conspirator	Angel	Executioner
Admirer	Aggressor	Drifter	Servant	King
Critic	Destroyer	Winner	Master	Queen
Waif	Victim	Loser	Savior	Prince
Abandoner	Avenger	Flunky	Monster	Princess
Caretaker	Leader	Clown	Child	Judge
Healer	Follower	Loner	Competitor	Examiner
Student	Rescuer	Partner	Pervert	Protege
Teacher	Hero	Arouser	Star	Mentor
Rival	Villain	Seducer	Mourner	
Explorer	Parent	Sinner		

Some adjectives

Destructive	Reassuring	Humiliated	Defeated	Dumb
Idealized	Scorned	Competent	Honored	Neglectful
Adoring	Scornful	Incompetent	Disgraced	Contaminated
Bereft	Bold	Worthwhile	Exalted	Empty
Lifeless	Cheerful	Pleasing	Degraded	Fragmented
Insulated	Engulfed	Superior	Rigid	Wounded
Abandoned	Large	Independent	Depleted	Dominant
Injured	Small	Withholding	Cooperative	Subordinate
Defective	Active	Passive	Rivalrous	Remote
Fragmented	Passive	Faulty	Frightened	Merging
Innocent	Good	Frantic	Needy	Pleasing
Anxious	Bad	Envious	Fragile	Noble
Cheerful	Weak	Disgusting	Faded	Vulgar
Glum	Needy	Pretty/handsome	Vengeful	Clean
Unappreciative	Duplicitous	Helpless	Uncertain	Dirty
Unavailable	Honest	Vain	Sexy	Caring
Responsible	Enraged	Incompetent	Coy	Cruel
Inadequate	Apologetic	Grudging	Devoted	Powerful
Grandiose	Vulnerable	Controlled	Merry	Flexible
Absent	Perfect	Triumphant	Aimless	Lost

Some useful combinations

Ambiguous critic	Helpless waif	Perfect performer
Scornful critic	Bereft child	Mutually engaged adult
Fooled critic	Worthless drifter	Sexually competent adult
Neglectful caretaker	Inadequate partner	Interested adult
Unreliable caretaker	Enraged victim	Competent (man, woman,
Withholding caretaker	Guilty wrongdoer	mother, father)
Impaired caretaker	Dulled loner	Compelling leader
Omnipotent caretaker	Repentant sinner	Special prince (princess)
Devoted caretaker	Heroic avenger	Uninteresting boy (girl)
Grandiose expert	As if devoted protegee	Wronged victim
Evil wrongdoer	Vulnerable student	Disgusting pervert
Defective wrongdoer	Passive follower	Engulfed subordinate
Insulated loner	Correct performer	Uncontrollable aggressor

**Table 11. Terms for Labeling Interpersonal Aims,
Intentions, and Expectations in Role Relationship Models**[a]

Attack, destroy, torture
Approach menacingly, scare
Express hostility
Angrily dismiss or reject
Starve, cut out, rip off, drain
Abandon, leave in lurch, reject, ignore
Neglect
Punish, take revenge
Be forgiven for misdeed
Delude, divert, mislead, deceive, trick to gain advantage
Accuse, blame, criticize
Put down, act superior to, scorn
Intrude upon, block, restrict
Enforce conformity, propriety
Manage, control, dominate
Benevolently monitor
Pamper, indulge
Cling to, depend on, partly merge with
Take in, learn from
Engage in logical and sensible analysis
Protect, back up
Provide for, nurture, support
Friendly engagement, mutuality, enduring attachment
Enjoy safe independence from
Admire, praise, endorse
Show off, exhibit, solicit self-centralized attention
Carefully and fairly consider, listen, show empathic understanding
Stroke, soothe, calm, warmly welcome, enjoy, entertain
Tenderly love, cherish, have sex with
Lustfully possess
Sadistically use
Masochistically submit
Possess totally
Engulf
Renounce possession of
Merge with
Compete with, beat
Be directed by
Wall off, insulate from
Use, manipulate as part of self

[a]Partially based on Benjamin (1979).

example is shown in Figure 6. In the *tra-la-la* state, Janice tried to feel and behave as if she were an active competent woman in a relationship with another active and competent person. The prototypical transaction was to be expression of mutual interest.

In the transition from the *tra-la-la* to a *hurt but working* state she gave up the self-concept of being competent, and experienced herself as having developmental difficulties. She could ask for help and continue to work because she felt she was continuing her personal development in the context of active engagement with a strong teacher or rescuer. She could remain in this state as long as she felt this relationship to be present.

Excerpt from the Third Therapy Hour

An example of the transition from the **self as active and competent** to the self as **impaired and willing to learn** is found in the following excerpt from the beginning of the third therapy session. She began in the *tra-la-la* state, with an animated and humorous imitation of what she planned to do.

The intent of this display was to capture the therapist's interest, and perhaps to test his willingness to converse socially rather than to work therapeutically with her on her difficulties. When she was convinced, for the moment, that the therapist was seriously interested in helping her, she changed to an interactional model in which she was like a student expressing her impairment (she stated that it upset her to "ooze" through her day) and expecting a teacher-rescuer type of response.

P: [Begins in *tra-la-la* style] Well, since last time, Doctor, [sniff] [dramatic play-acting] I, I find myself storing up things to tell you but, you know, things that happen or things that I think about a lot or something, so, tsk, hm [play-acting] I'll have to tell him this. [She pauses. The therapist listens quietly and intently. She becomes more nervous as she enters a *hurt but working* state.] I'm not sure why; whether I think you'll be interested, or whether I think it's relevant. Whether it's something I want to work out. There's **something** I'd like to work out; [pause, continues in *hurt but working* style] it happened, has been happening, guess it's still heavy [cough]. I got **really, really** depressed last week. I don't know what day it started and I couldn't really put a reason to it. You know, no incident, nothing happened. I wasn't thinking any train of thought and suddenly I just [pause] got depressed. And, uh [long pause] just [pause] it lasted for days and I would kind of—I was just sort of half functioning at work, hm, ttst, I can't think of a word, oozing my way through the day, and I managed to do a couple of wrong things and [sigh] I'm really upset about that.

The role relationship between **impaired learner** and **strong teacher** was tolerable and somewhat desirable. But it held threats and was hard to stabilize. As already discussed, she entered it when she gave up, or was urged to give up, the pretense of being fully competent **and** when support was available.

As shown in Figure 7, she also tended to go beyond it by exaggerating the traits of each character. The weaker role of the **learner** rather than the **competent complete woman** could be extended into experiencing herself as too **weak** in relation to another more **powerful** person. The **teacher** could be seen as more than a source of ideas or a partial role model, and became the principal supplier of her sense of identity. This is the role relationship that characterized one of the internal experiences when she felt *acute self-disgust*. The prototypical situation was the unresolved issue of her relationship with her mother. She felt self-disgust when she saw herself assuming her mother's identity, becoming a defective extension of her mother rather than a fully independent person. The threat of entering the *self-disgust* state motivated her to resume the **competent self-concept** of the *tra-la-la* state rather than to remain with the **impaired but learning self-images** of the *hurt but working* state. She would resume these **competent self-images**, and so change state, whenever she had made some gain (as in learning something from a teacher) or when she could successfully defend against the "news" about herself that led to the impaired self-concepts (see Figure 6).

Obtaining supplies, even learning from someone, was dangerous in another way. Taking from someone could be seen as being too strong as well as too weak. To learn from another could mean to absorb too strongly and too much. She feared a state in which she would behave like a vampire and deplete the other person who gave too much. This concept rested on a primitive belief that psychological supplies such as care were limited and so could be exhausted. It could also rest on a covert family belief in which her mother felt she had given so much that if Janice now went away from her, she would feel depleted and misused. In addition, the transition to this state was fostered by a wish within Janice to reverse roles from her relatively weak position to that of a stronger person who subjugated someone else. To avoid the feared *acute self-disgust and guilt* outcome of the "taking" kind of interpersonal relationship in the *hurt but working* state, she tended to revert to the *tra-la-la* state. This model of the role relationships that underlie common state transitions is shown in Figure 7.

To recapitulate, Janice might oscillate from the *hurt but working* state back to the *tra-la-la* state under several conditions: (1) when she could no longer tolerate the concept of self-impairment, (2) when she was in

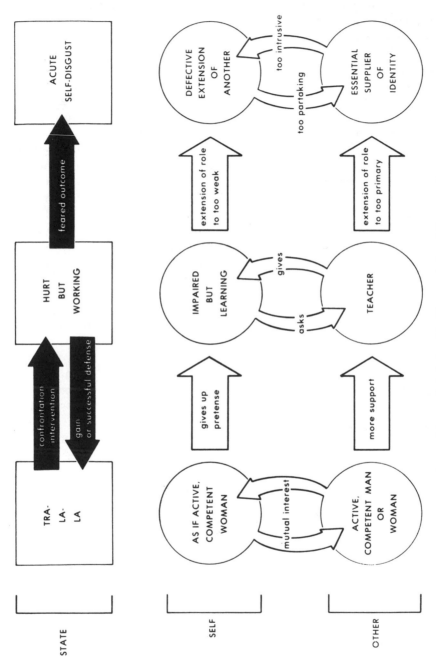

Figure 6. A Format for Modeling Role Relationship Characteristics of Common State Transitions.

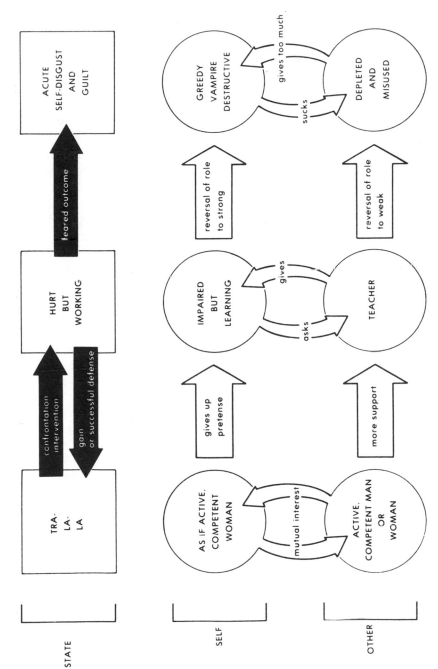

Figure 7. Main Role Relationships for the *Tra-la-la, Hurt but Working,* and *Acute Self-Disgust and Guilt* States.

danger of seeing herself as taking too much from a rescuing or helping person, and (3) when she successfully avoided contemplating the information about herself that diminished her self-esteem.

The *hurt and not working* state has already been characterized by an activated self-schema in which she needed much but expected nothing and so fed herself. This was a state of withdrawal in which the other person was viewed as unworthy, withholding, or lost. There was an illusion of self-sufficiency, as if she were a cocoon (Modell, 1975). If another person entered during this state, she shifted from withdrawal into herself as the sole object of her concern to interest in the other as a potential source of support. This led to a *crying* state, if such a display of emotion attracted help. There was, however, a feared outcome: She might cry and find no one present. This led to a state of *acute self-disgust* in which she experienced herself as weak, wounded, and in need of a person who had been lost to her. These transitions are diagrammed in Figure 8.

Not diagrammed in Figure 8 is a *crying* state that also led to a *play-acting* state in which she only pretended to be crying, a variant of the *tra-la-la* state. This fooled the person trying to rescue her, and whom she then regarded with contempt. When she saw herself fooling another person, she was also in danger of feelings of self-contempt for taking things she did not really need. Worse yet, she might fool someone into thinking that she was really not needy. This person would then desert her. Because she was really needy, she would again be deprived.

Another set of self-schemata organized some states of *acute self-disgust and shame*. She was vulnerable to self-concepts as defective or guilty in relationship to a strong, superior, critical judge. One example was her feeling of being accused of sexual misdeeds by her mother: "I try to justify myself . . . . Like she's [her mother] sitting up there judging me. And saying, 'You're a slut, you're a nymphomaniac.'" This state, hard for her pride to tolerate, quickly changes, as shown in Figure 9. A common shift was projection of possibly bad traits onto the another person, with reversal of their roles. She assumed the role of superior judge, criticizing the other as a wrongdoer or a person more defective than she. The *competitive* state that resulted was a struggle between them over who was to blame or who was most defective. This *competitive* state was unstable because she feared her own destructiveness; her rage might destroy the other. She could then ward off the danger of guilt and an acute self-disgust state by another reversal of roles. She would shift back to seeing herself as the person who was not vulnerable. Another way out was, when possible, to resume the self-images and self-displays that characterized the *tra-la-la* state.

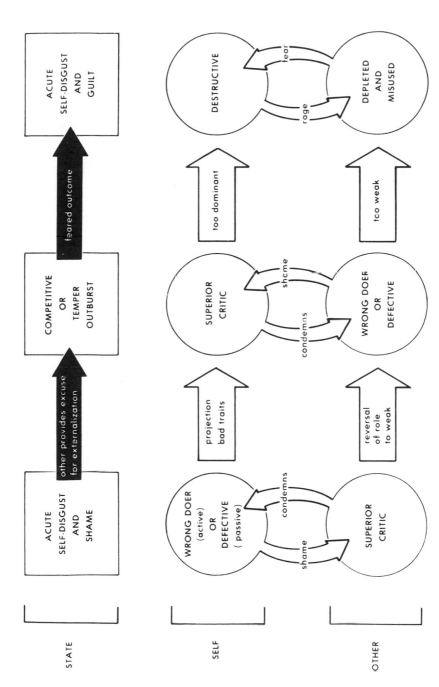

Figure 8. Role Relationships for the *Acute Self-Disgust and Shame, Competitive,* and *Acute Self-Disgust and Guilt* States.

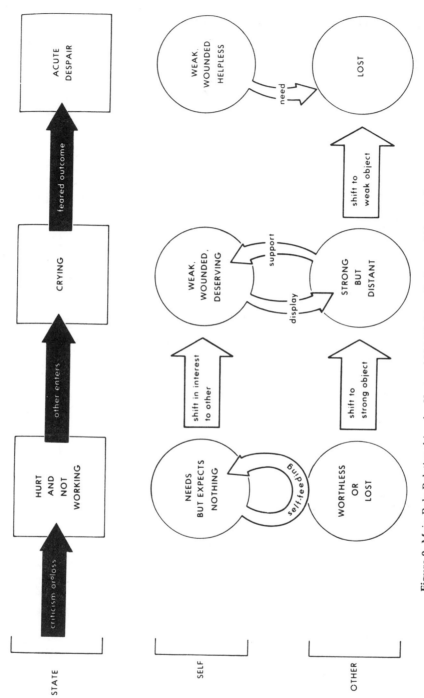

Figure 9. Main Role Relationships for *Hurt and Not Working*, *Crying*, and *Despair* States.

While Figures 6, 7, 8, and 9 do not examine all possibilities, they do indicate the most important roles of self and other. These role relationships can be summarized as they relate to states and the earlier list of common self-concepts found in Table 7. The result is Table 12, which includes an underachieved, longed-for state of intimate sharing. Adding desired and ideal states and role relationship models conveys the wishful component of motivation.

Such tables are open-ended. For example, Table 12 summarizes Janice as far as the information available from the brief therapy led to an understanding of some patterns. Many of the dyads shown could be seen as variants of her relationship around giving and taking supplies and being connected with or independent from her mother. The relationship with her father did not surface as extensively during this period of therapy. Undoubtedly a repertoire of dyads and triads would involve him and significant others during her development. But such information was not available. Had she been seen in a more extensive therapy, such data would have allowed the list to become broader, deeper, and clearer (for an example, see Horowitz, 1987, in press).

Wishes, Threats, and Defenses. A dynamic triangle of wishes, threats or fears, and coping or defensive compromises can be modeled at every

Table 12. Complementary Roles of Self and Other as They Relate to States

State	Recurrent self-concepts	Complementary concepts of other
Intimate sharing (unachieved ideal)	Competent	Competent
Tra-la-la	As if competent	Competent
Hurt but working	Impaired but learning student	Teacher
Hurt and not working	Needy but self-sufficient and self-feeding	Lost, worthless, or remote
Crying	Needy and deserving	Rescuer
Competitive	Wrongly accused, critic	Wrongdoer or defective
Acute self-disgust	Defective extension of another	Supplier of identity
	Wrongdoer	Superior critic
	Greedy, selfish	Depleted and misused
	Depleted and misused	Greedy, selfish
	Depleted and helpless	Lost

level of configurational analysis. At this step, the role relationship models provide a useful component for this purpose. A Defensive Organization Format permits a systematic approval that contains places for desired and feared states (the middle sections of Table 13), and either symptomatic or nonsymptomatic avoidances (at the top and bottom, as problematic and compromise states, of Table 13).

Scripts, Schematic Agendas, and Story Lines

The aim here is to describe prominent, repetitive interpersonal behavioral patterns as they are based on inner patterns. To do so, one describes the organization of shifts in roles or actions in terms of patterned sequences. One form for this is to fill in the blanks of this mapping sentence: "If (I, he, she, they, it) _____ then it will follow that (I, he, she, they, it) will _____ because _____. Note that the "because" point adds other types of schemata, those of enduring attitudes, values, or causal belief systems.

For Janice, one could report this for both regressive dependent aims and progressive independent ones. For example, one sequence would be to give up identification with her mother as a self-denying, giving, but depleted caretaker and decide to be a competent, independent career

Table 13. A Defensive Organizational Format: Including Wishes, Fears, Compromises, and Symptom Formation at the Person Schemata Level

	Self	Aims	Other
Problem state *Hurt and not* *working*	Needy but expects nothing	None	Worthless or lost
Dreaded state *Acute self-disgust* *and guilt*	Destructive vampire ←───	Takes and hurts ──→ Exposes harm done to evoke guilt	Depleted and misused
Desired state *Intimate sharing*	Competent, crea- tive woman ←───	Mutual give and ──→ take	Competent companion
Compromise state *Tra-la-la*	As if competent woman ←───	Self-display ───→ Interest	Competent companion

woman. A positive sequence is: "If I become a skilled person then it will follow that I will get respect because 'they' value competence." A negative sequence is: "If I become a skilled person then it will follow that my mother will feel bad because she does not wish to be surpassed by a female member of the family such as her own daughter." By description of sequences one moves toward formulation of both scripts and relationship conflicts.

Relationship Conflicts

The description of relationship conflicts may begin with notes about personal aims that seem to cause repeated problems because of the anticipated consequences. As these are elaborated, it will be possible to fill out a Conflictual Relationship Schematization Form. This provides a model of conflicts and/or deficiencies surrounding the personal agenda of the individual at the present "existential crisis" or "life developmental moment." Several forms might be filled out for different thematic conflicts.

The Conflictual Relationship Schematization Form allows conflicted aims to be worked out in progressive and regressive forms. Only portions of the form may be filled out, depending on what inferences can be drawn from the available data. Thus, if information is available, describe the developmental basis for these role relationship models. Relate shifts in self-concept to recent life events, changes in social context, or physical occurrences.

Janice, in her 20s, still faces the life task of solidification of her own independence and patterns of affiliation to others. She had left home only months before the death of a brother resulted in a return for the funeral, and a reactivation of the idea of remaining with her family. Throughout adolescence she had experienced strong wishes to become a different kind of person from the woman whose role her mother extolled, exemplified, yet complained about. Janice acted in a manner counter to this role but felt inauthentic, as if it was an artifice to avoid mimicry of her mother, and not a true path for herself.

The two aspects of the ambivalent attachment to her mother were reflected in many of her statements: "When I think now, and I think maybe that's what I wanted, you know, like you reach out, you loop each other's hands, and you look into each other's eyes. And, you know, something has passed between you [her and her mother]." The other side of her ambivalence, related to the funeral for her brother, was also expressed: "I remember crying on one night, a night or so after I came home. Getting really mad at my mother and going upstairs and starting to cry out of anger."

The format for interpersonal conflict themes developed by Luborsky (1984) is shown in Table 14. Putting the entries for Janice into outline form, a core conflictual relationship theme is as follows:

> Wish: I want to go ahead and form my own life autonomously from my mother even though my brother has died and she has asked me to return home, but the consequences would be
> 1. Negative response from objects: My mother will be hurt by this separation.
> 2. Negative response from self: Because I leave my mother, I will feel frightened and not up to the tasks of working, living alone, and making new attachments.
> 3. Positive response from object: She will appreciate me for my productivity and successful development.

Table 14. Format for the Core Conflictual Relationship Theme Formulation[a]

Wishes, needs, intentions	Consequences
	Negative response from object
	a. _____
	b. _____
	c. _____
	Negative response from self
	a. _____
	b. _____
	c. _____
W: "I wish from object":	Positive response from object
A. (General) _____	a. _____
i. (Specific) _____	b. _____
ii. (Specific) _____	c. _____
iii. (Specific) _____	Positive response from self
B. (General) _____	a. _____
i. (Specific) _____	b. _____
	c. _____

[a]Types of components are listed in order with the most frequent first (from Luborsky, 1984).

4. Positive response from self: I will feel authentic, useful, and competent and so can love myself, and stop feeling self-disgusted.

The Conflictual Relationship Schematization Format (CRSF) shown in Table 15 models not only the conflict of progressive aims, as just indicated above, but the conflict involving the threats of regressive arms, as well as the conflict *between* regressive and progressive aims. Janice wishes autonomy (progressive aim); she also wishes a return to dependency (going backwards, hence regressive). One goal competes with another. Thus, within the Conflictual Relationship Schematization Format (CRSF), or in prose statements at this point, one can describe four types of conflict around a given relationship theme. These are the conflicts between wish and threat, regressive and progressive strivings, positive and negative consequences of potential acts upon wishes, and the internal or external sources of consequences. To illustrate:

1. *Wish versus Threat*
   The wish for autonomy from her mother might lead to separation acts that hurt her mother so badly that Janice would feel too guilty, or might lead to being so isolated when apart from her mother that she would feel too lonely.
2. *Progressive versus Regressive Aims*
   The aim for autonomy is opposed by Janice's wish to return home to her mother.
3. *Positive versus Negative Consequences*
   If Janice accepts her mother's appeal to return home as a consequence of the funeral for Janice's brother, she gains the connection with her mother (gratifying the dependent wish), BUT she gives up the chance to establish herself in another city and may become anxious over a smothering degree of closeness.

Table 15. Conflictional Relationship Schematization Format (CRSF) for Themes

Progressive conflict	Regressive conflict
1. Wish	1. Wish
Impediments to aim	Impediments to aim
2. Fear	2. Fear
3. Defense	3. Defense
4. Outcome	4. Outcome

4. *External versus Internal*

> If Janice returns home, her mother will feel better for the reunion, but Janice will suffer from giving up her effort at autonomy at a crucial time, when she has not yet mastered the life transition to a career and a relationship or family of her own generation.

The above conflicts are the ordinary dilemmas of life. Everyone has to make these choices. In neurotic conflict each horn of the dilemma has a high degree of anxiety and so choices are avoided or undone. This may be because the neurotic has rigid agendas and scripts that do not allow flexible use of one or another role relationship model. Instead, the neurotic has to repeat a long but inconclusive sequence. The neurotic confluence of progressive and regressive relationship scripts for Janice is shown in Table 16. I think it is worth reading both vertically and horizontally. It contains a lot of information in an organized way and could provide the "big picture" of what is clarified and interpreted in a psychotherapy.

DEVELOPMENT

Having described current relationship patterns, person schemata, scripts, and conflicts, one can then attempt to describe historical developments of the key features. Whether or not this can be done depends on how much historical information is available and what can be reconstructed. This information was not available in the illustration used here, but a psychoanalytic case is reported elsewhere and shows one method of organizing such developmental information (Horowitz, 1977a, in press). The particular person and the purposes of the configurational analysis will indicate whether to focus on the present, to carry these models through several past generations, to focus on small or large group patterns, or to separate person schemata into further subclassifications.

SUMMARY

In order to describe a person's relationship patterns, it is necessary to accept the concept that everyone has many schemata, both persisting and fluctuating agendas, and motives that may conflict at conscious and unconscious levels of operation. A useful beginning is the development of a simple list of self-concepts. Supplementary elaboration will expand

Table 16. Conflictional Relationship Schematization Format (CRSF)
for Janice
Theme: Direction of Self and Relationship with Mother

Progressive conflict	Regressive conflict
1. **Wish** Autonomy from her mother	1. **Wish** Dependence upon her mother for identity, connection, and life direction
Impediments to aim Death of brother is demoralizing, she feels too alone in a city far from home, her career skills are not fully developed	**Impediments to aim** None; mother is encouraging her to do it
2. **Fear** May try and fail, be scorned by others, and feel self-critical (anxiety over loss of status) If succeeds, will feel has hurt mother by surpassing her (anxiety over guilt)	2. **Fear** Will scorn self as weak, lazy, and defective (anxiety over shame) Will get anxious that too close (anxiety over merger)
3. **Defense** If too anxious, shift to regressive aim If too anxious, inhibit contemplation of her life plans If too anxious, challenge the competency of others	3. **Defense** If too anxious, shift to progressive aims If too anxious, inhibit memory of brother's death, funeral, mother's wish for her If too anxious, criticize mother or those who are like mother
4. **Outcome** Impairment at work, near to being fired for staying home Indecision on advancing skills needed for career, states of *acute self-disgust* and *guilt* warded off by self-stabilization in *hurt and not working* state	4. **Outcome** Inhibition of mourning of brother Fear of entry into *intimate sharing* state, attempts to stabilize the *tra-la-la* state in order to get some relationship support without the danger of intimacy

and revise this list. The self-experiences overtly or symbolically contained in the states of mind in which problems occur will often provide the first entries.

Self-concepts can be further elaborated as complements to recurrent views of others. The role relationships that emerge can be depicted as models of two persons, three persons, or small group situations. Modeling key conflicts will be especially useful. The control operations that decide, in effect, when to change the currently dominant organizing schemata should then be considered. This is the purpose of the next step.

CHAPTER FOUR

Ideas, Emotions, and Controls

Step 4. Information Processing: *As a point of departure, take from the problem list repetitive intrusions and omissions from rational consciousness. Model central themes of conflict as constellations of ideas, emotions, and maneuvers of control over modes of representing and communicating thought and feeling. Include wishes, threats, and defenses.*

Invariably, a human problem is embedded in a matrix of important personal and social meanings. Processing, and controlling the processing of this information, will often be the cause of changes from one state to another. This step will deal with descriptions of meanings and processing patterns.

Any situation, whether it is caused by internal or external changes, involves a network much like that of a large, busy city from which many roads emerge; various lines of meaning extend from the event and follow diverse paths. Even when a single problem is the focus, several thematic constellations of ideas, feelings, and controls may be described. Any moment in a life carries with it needs, demands, chances for displeasure or for pleasure, for gratification or for harm. Each person brings to these moments his habitual styles of knowing, thinking, reacting, deciding, and acting. All of these processes are part of the constellation of meaning.

Very often, the constellations of meaning selected for analysis at such points in time will consist of lines of association and decision making that have been disrupted, or at least interrupted. Significant events produce fear of harm or anxiety about opportunities that might be missed. These events set in motion streams of consciousness that in turn produce unpleasant feeling states. To stop or to avoid these states, the forward process of thought may be altered or derailed. A significant event, how-ever, carries new information into mental activity. The information must be processed in order to bring inner models into alignment with the reality of shifts in the situation.

Even when the route to completed processing of information is blocked, stymied, or interrupted, relevant constellations of ideas and feelings are retained in some sort of memory, where ideas are warded off rather than lost. These ideas and feelings contain a powerful property for repetition. I find it useful to call this a completion tendency (Horo-witz, 1986). Even though the person attempts to prevent conscious expressions, the ideas and feelings emerge intrusively. When there is not an intrusive return, they may nevertheless occur in disguised and symbolic form or influence decisions without conscious recognition of such effects. The struggle between aims at expression of these ideas and efforts to avoid the emotional threat of such expression is sometimes called an impulse-defense configuration. Such constellations will be described here.

BACKGROUND

The concept of emotionally powerful, conflictual, and warded-off sets of ideas (or "complexes") reflects the contributions to dynamic psy-chiatry made by Charcot (1877), Janet (1965), and Breuer and Freud (1895/1957). Traumatic life events occurred and led to what Freud (1920/1955b) called untamed memories. These memories and associated ideas were not dormant; instead, they had an intrinsic tendency to return to mind with an intrusive and emotionally intense quality. The emotional responses were seen by Freud as due to accumulated undischarged excitations and to the incompatibility between ideas associated with the traumatic event and other mental attitudes.

Freud conceptualized as quasi-instinctual the powerful factors that led to the return of warded-off ideas to consciousness and called this tendency the repetition compulsion. He proposed that the compulsion to repeat was counteracted by defensive operations such as repression. The interaction between warded-off but dynamically powerful ideas and defensive maneuvers led in an immediate sense to symptoms, and in the long run, to pathological character traits.

The concept of signal anxiety incorporated a feedback component to this model (Freud, 1926/1959b; Rangell, 1968). That is, information processing continued unconsciously, or at periphery of awareness. The incompatible ideas were appraised, and recognition of their incompatibility led to anxiety. Freud called this type of emotional anxiety response a signal because the emotion itself carried information about the threat that might occur if these ideas reached awareness or motivated action. Signal anxiety was then formulated as the motive for instigation of defensive processes. By this theory Freud also explained how therapy progressed by (1) making the warded-off ideas and feelings conscious, (2) working through conflicted aims and meanings by conscious assessment and communication, (3) improving modulation or control of conflicts, and (4) releasing or discharging excitations. The concept of working through was described as allowing rational thought and problem solving to take place, processes by which the incompatibilities between sets of ideas could be reduced.

Attempts to shorten the period of time required for psychoanalytic treatment focused on working on specific sectors of ideation. Ferenczi (1926/1950), Rank (1929), and Alexander and French (1946) were prominent in describing such focal and time-limited therapeutic work. A central task was defining, early in treatment, key conflicts upon which to focus. Balint, Ornstein, and Balint (1972), Caplan (1961), Sifneos (1972), Mann (1973), Malan (1976a), and Horowitz, Marmar, Krupnick et al. (1984) have carried these ideas further into descriptions of brief therapy techniques, where the focus is on working through current crises and central conflicts. The development of models of key ideational conflicts has also been shaped by the revolution in information processing and decision theory (Peterfreund, 1971; Thickstun and Rosenblatt, 1977; Erdelyi, 1984; Edelson, 1984; Eagle, 1984).

PREVIOUS METHODS FOR OUTLINING IDEATIONAL CONSTELLATIONS

Some of the background methods outlined in the previous chapter for describing core interpersonal fantasies tended to condense concepts that are separated here. For example, the Luborsky system for the CCRT presents not only a role relationship model but a train of thought: "I would like to leave my mother but I am unsure if I can be competent on my own." Klein (1967) has offered a system more purely related to the flow of ideas. He simply diagrams the sequential flow and feedback relations of repetitive ideas.

Another approach is that of using a content analysis manual to encourage clinical judges to decipher, according to common formats, a given patient's "unconscious plan." Weiss (1967, 1972; Weiss, Sampson, and Caston, 1977), and Weiss and Sampson (1986) have suggested that persons, even in conflict, have an intended program. Working in collaboration with them, Caston (1977) developed a manual for "plan diagnosis" that uses several main headings to outline relevant patterns to be described. The first heading asks for the goals of the person. This heading can be subdivided further into immediate and eventual goals, which can best be stated by means of concrete examples. Since these examples are usually interpersonal themes and issues of self-competence, the system resembles the method of Luborsky (1984). The second heading is also similar to that of Luborsky; it consists of a statement of the principal obstacles to the plan. The third heading describes the means to be used when the plan is set into motion. Two other divisions involve the therapy process and will be discussed later. As in the Luborsky system, the plan diagnosis system leads to a relatively unitary statement that compresses together relationships **structures** and ideational **processes**.

SUGGESTED METHODS FOR FORMULATING THE PROCESSING OF IDEATIONAL CONSTELLATIONS

The model to be described follows the traditional route of dynamic formulation in that it aims toward statement of what ideas and feelings are warded off when they tend to emerge, why they press for expression in terms of anticipated gains, why they are warded off in terms of potential threats, and how they are warded off. One problem with such formulations has been to discover a way to go beyond the content of the warded-off themes to a description of the processes of interaction between events, ideas, emotions, and controls. The interaction between these processes sometimes makes prose descriptions of them difficult; clarification can be achieved through the use of diagrams.

The format for such diagrams relates the meanings of events to the associations they evoke, and to the inner models or structures of meaning, the self-images and role relationships described in the previous chapter. This format allows clear illustration of the relationship between these sets of ideas and emotional reactions they elicit, and permits examination of conscious and unconscious aspects of these processes (Horowitz, 1977b, 1986).

The basic principle of the format is to model conflict as the discrepancy that arises during a process of comparison between sets of ideas. The discrepancy may be among sets of new ideas, among sets of enduring attitudes, or between new ideas and enduring attitudes. **In** this format emotional processes are recorded as a signaling system announcing the degree and quality of these discrepancies. These emoting processes add information and that information may result in changed states. In addition, the arousal of feeling motivates controls that, in feedback, affect the continued processing of information. Change in controls changes ideas and feelings, and so states change. In other words, control operations regulate states by altering the play of ideas and emotional responses (see Figure 10). If the overall play of controls increases adaptation, then the global regulatory maneuver is called a coping operation. If the controls aim to avoid danger, but in turn cause some lack of adaptation or some maladaptive behavior, the maneuver is called a defensive operation. In the event that the controls do not function, the situation is called an adaptive failure (Haan, 1977; Horowitz, 1986).

In Figure 10, the inciting occurrence is called an event, an action, or an active memory of an event. An example of the latter would be

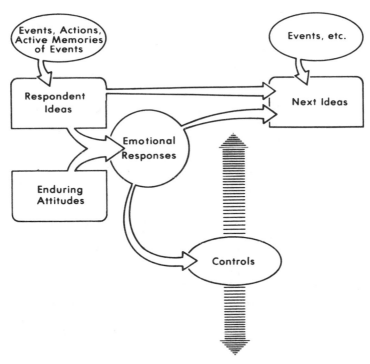

Figure 10. Thematic Progression Form for Diagramming the Sequential and Simultaneous Interaction of Events, Ideas, Emotions, and Controls.

recollection of a fearsome situation such as a death, even though that event had taken place sometime in the past. An inciting event, one that leads into the format, would also include "internal events." That is, the onset selected for a model might be a sudden impulse, a daydream, a dream or nightmare, or even a bodily sensation such as pain, tension, or palpitations. The inciting event is any stimulus that requires interpretation of meanings, any circumstance that elicits a variety of associations. These are the respondent ideas shown in Figure 10. To another person, these associations may seem relevant or irrelevant, realistic or unrealistic. To the subject, fantasy meanings or incorrect generalizations may be as important as realistic appraisals. Such fantasy meanings must be included in our models because they have important motivational properties.

These varied associative responses to events couple with the event to create a constellation of ideas that is matched with relatively enduring inner models such as self-images, role relationship schemata, body images, maps of the person's world, and basic plans for behavior. When the "news" does not match with existing models or expectations, emotion is aroused. These emotional responses are processes expressed in psychological and physiological form, and, as mentioned, they in turn are sensed as events and represented as ideas.

These processes and expressions influence controls. **If the response is pleasure, if things look better than existing models or expectations, control efforts are aimed at continuation or amplification of the state by facilitation of the impressions. If the response is displeasure, control efforts aim at altering the state by inhibiting, derailing, or deranging the impressions.**

To further understand these abstract statements, consider a serious stressful life event such as the death of a loved one. Were "ideal" information processing to take place, the person would appraise the loss realistically and, based on this appraisal, plan the most constructive line of response, including the expectation of his own period of mourning. Whatever the final situation, inner models would be aligned with external realities by the necessary changes in such conceptual structures of meaning as self-concepts and role relationship models (Lazarus and Folkman, 1984; Janis, 1969; Horowitz, 1986). The perceived difference between the serious life event, the death of a loved one, and the inner model of the previously enduring relationship is what makes the life event "serious" and "stressful." This difference sets in motion thought processes directed at understanding the implications of the loss for the past, the present, and the future.

The realization of the discrepancy, however, also evokes emotions such as grief, panic, fear, and resentment, which act as threats. To avoid the threat of an increase or continuation of these emotions, and especially to avoid the danger of intolerable levels of feeling, the process of recognition of implications is regulated. Complete recognition of the power of the loss would be intolerable. Total nonrecognition would be unrealistic and therefore nonadaptive. Gradual, step-by-step dosing of recognition would be a normal process. One can model the status of ideas and feelings, of various associated trains of thoughts about the past and future, at each point in the process.

The relevant experiences of a given person provide the point of departure for plotting the components in this format. This clarifies the reasons for the entry of the person into problem states and the processes that cause state transitions. Changes can be described as alteration in contents, in the relative status of varied premises, as shifts in quality or intentionality of expression, and in the linkage between sets of ideas and feelings. Change can also be described in terms of altered forms of representation, accessibility to conscious reflection, organizational styles, ways of perceiving, and decision-making capacities. In short, contents may change, forms may change, and formation of processes may change.

When there is one set, or several sets, of important but warded-off ideas, they should be included as part of the focus on informational issues. In order to gather information about such sets of ideas, it is usually necessary to review the entire therapy process, not just data from initial evaluation and treatment sessions. One can then clarify how the contents were warded off—or confronted—for the period before therapy began.

While this text focuses on psychological factors, biological factors should be included whenever pertinent. For example, a toxic disturbance may make complex organization of information impossible or unstable. Description of information processing in such an instance would include statement of the cognitive operations the person could not perform, the maneuvers used as substitutes, and the capacities that remained intact.

SUBCLASSIFICATIONS IN STEP 4

The summary of Step 4 given at the head of this chapter may now be fleshed out in terms of how to formulate both current themes and habitual styles of processing information.

Step 4A. *Themes*

4A (1). Indicate major constellations of memories and fantasies as composites of ideas, feelings, and actions that influence current states of mind, especially those related to the symptomatic phenomena described in Step 1 and the problem states described in Step 2. Describe memory and fantasy formats that are repetitive and related to the phenomena of Step 1 and the states of Step 2. Describe trains of thought that are initiated by wishes or needs and activate the problematic and dreaded self- and object concepts described in Step 3. Relate these constellations to recent life events, to environmental or physiological conditions or deficiencies, and to social support systems.

4A (2). Derive a model of the degree to which outer reality accords with the subject's conscious views, assumptions, and unconscious organizing schematizations, including self-concepts and role relationship models. Indicate how discrepancies between outer world and inner assumptions, inner motives, and inner critical or moral assessments evoke emotional responses and lead the subject to self-regulations and entry into various expressive or defensive states of mind.

4A (3). Derive a model of how control operations influence the processing of themes consciously and unconsciously, using the Thematic Progression Form to interrelate events, reactive ideas, enduring beliefs, emotional and response potentials, and controls (see Figure 10).

4A (4). If information is available, indicate why progression toward completion of a train of thought, emotional working through, or decision making is blocked for each theme, noting the developmental basis for the blockage and the potential course to take toward resolution.

Step 4B. *Habitual Styles*

Indicate the subject's typical use of specific information-processing strategies and how this leads to idiosyncratic use of any specific mode of expression, defensive operation, and/or coping strategy. Relate different modes for processing or representing information to different states of mind noted in Step 2. (For a classification of coping and defensive operations, see also Horowitz, 1986, pp. 101–110; Haan, 1977; Vaillant, 1977.)

Themes can be examined by selecting a repetitive and important idea and articulating an associational tree out of the current variations. These limbs include relevant memories and fantasies from the past and the extension of the themes into the projected future. For example, if a patient reported a recurrent fantasy, memory, hallucination, or delusion, one could start with the contents, piece together the meanings, and describe the process of forming the experience (Horowitz, 1983).

Premises, as recently pointed out by Beck (1985), are of a more general order than thoughts; they operate at a preconscious level as automatically functioning rules and injunctions about how to make decisions. The basic premises can be described and related to the relationship between situations, ideas, themes, and styles of solution to problems. Describing the associational matrix of important, warded-off, or intrusive ideas is usually impossible when working only with the information known early in a treatment. Similarly, guiding premises are usually known only later. That is why, in a review of a change process already completed, all the data are examined and organized in terms of the status of information at treatment entry.

RECAPITULATION

Despite the possible complexity of this step, the first approach should be a bold statement of constellations of ideas that are either warded off or repetitively intrusive in relation to conscious thought and action. A good place to start will usually be found in the lists of problems and states. An attempt should be made to infer why such ideas are currently active and why efforts at their control are made. These control efforts should themselves be described and related to the person in terms of habit patterns or novel (even creative) approaches to conflicts. Emotional responses, as well as ideas and actions that might occur without adequate control, should be added to indicate motivations.

ILLUSTRATION

Janice was depressed because her life was not going well, and she wished to examine this problem conceptually. Her main entry complaint, however, was that she sensed she was not reacting to the recent death of her brother, and her visit home for the funeral, in a beneficial way. She was preoccupied with this recent serious event but the funeral and death led to asociative meanings that she was warding off. She experienced intrusive beginnings of a thought cycle but interrupted the cycle before the ideas and feelings could reach a point of resolution.

This overall constellation can be divided into three subsidiary sets. One was her reaction to the loss of her brother. A second was her reaction to the visit home, the idea of returning home for good, and a confrontation with the meaning of deciding to continue her life away from home. A third was her reaction to her "silly" behavior when she was at home for the funeral. The loss of her brother had to result in mourning. She was still in a phase of denial of the reality of the event as the end of a relationship, and its implications for her own vulnerability to death or injury. Because of her existing susceptibility to depression and apathy, and other priorities existing in her life, she avoided confrontation with these and other themes of grief work, felt no grief, and castigated herself about its absence. The particular therapy period under examination focused not so much on this mourning subtheme as on the more emergent issues of the independence–dependence theme, and her reaction to her "silly" behavior at the funeral. Therefore, these themes will be used in what follows as primary illustrations. It should be noted, however, that a mourning process was initiated during therapy, and continued in the posttherapy period.

A second subtheme was used as one of the main illustrations in the previous chapter. It had to do with the symbolic meaning of returning home and her responses to her mother's request that now, in view of the death of her brother, she might return home from a life that her mother considered improper. The symbolic meaning of being separated one step further from her family by the loss of her brother, the idea that she too could be vulnerable if away from home, and the confrontation with her own appraisal of her current life course were all associated. The continuation of this theme was to think through how best to effect her separation from her home, and her next steps for continued independence, but she warded off these ideas. Despite such avoidances, however, she remained preoccupied with these issues. That is, these topics tended to return to awareness in symbolic form as intrusive episodes of acute self-disgust.

The reasons for preoccupation with this theme and repetition of it had to do with anticipated gains. If she could plan for continued development of her personal competency, for stabilization of well-being while away from home by new mature attachments to others, then she could hope to become a mature woman, one who could feel authentic and self-loving rather than self-disgusted. If she were to remain in limbo, neither dependent nor independent, or if she were to return home, then she would never measure up to her own personal ideals, and her self-esteem and interpersonal gratifications would suffer.

Despite the anticipated gains of working it through, the theme was warded off whenever it repeated itself because the ideas themselves led to painful emotional states. If Janice left her mother, she would have to tolerate both feeling bad over hurting her mother's feelings and the anxiety of separate living. When she examined her present state of incomplete competency for independent living she felt acute self-disgust, as she did when she contemplated surrendering to fantasies of returning home. She used a variety of avoidance techniques to elude the threat of such states of self-disgust, as well as the humiliation involved in communicating these ideas to others. She attempted to inhibit the emergence of these ideas; when this was unsuccessful, she used generalization and intellectualization to keep the issue at a vague, impersonal, and hence unemotional level. When it became necessary, she supplemented these inhibitory maneuvers by switching attitudes, undoing statements, and reversing roles. When reversing roles she externalized threatening traits from herself to others.

Her own behavior at the funeral provided another memory that was difficult to integrate. She felt that in a social sense she had not mourned appropriately; she had not cried enough. She contrasted herself with her mother, who cried a great deal. In addition, she had withdrawn to her room and read, instead of participating in family gatherings. Her mother rebuked her for her "silliness" (behaving in an inappropriately joking manner during this time) and for her withdrawal.

She would tend to remember these because by thinking them over she could eventually work through the memories and lay them to rest. For example, she could have decided for herself, in retrospect, what behavior had been appropriate and what had been inappropriate. If she felt remorse for her acts she could have forgiven herself, planned to do better in the future, apologized, or performed some other act of contrition. After thinking through the implications, making up her mind, planning and executing action, reorganizing her self- and world picture, she could have been **done** with this life event and moved on to other tasks. But she was conflicted in this situation; it is important in this step to describe that conflict as simply as possible.

Janice warded off potential self-rebuke for her immature behavior at the funeral, her yearning to return home to her mother, and her guilt at leaving once again through a variety of defenses. As already noted, she **inhibited** the flow of thinking that would be set in motion by the memory. She used **intellectualization** and **generalization** to avoid direct awareness of her own desires to return home, and her own self-criticism. In communicative contexts, when ideas became too foreboding, she **switched** from one attitude to another in her assertion of self-attributes. For example, she might follow a phrase that demonstrated her weakness in a situation with another phrase that indicated her strength, one indicating her subordination with one indicating her assertiveness. In doing so, she would also **exchange roles** with the other person. Furthermore, she could **externalize** attributes, talking of others as selfish when she was approaching conscious ideas about her own selfishness.

These avoidance maneuvers were a general pattern. That is, her habitual cognitive and communicative style in states of conflict included inhibition, vagueness, disavowal of ideas, and switching between opposite attitudes. These can now be illustrated for the overall theme that, for the sake of brevity, will be called the **homesickness theme** in what follows.

Excerpt from the First Therapy Hour

In the first therapy session inhibition and disavowal were present, as when she gratuitously said, "I don't get homesick," and in the next hour repeated, "Did I tell you I don't get homesick? That I don't miss my family and my friends? . . . Why don't I miss them?" These and several other habitual control maneuvers are illustrated in the following more detailed interchange taken from the first hour of therapy:

P: She [her girl friend] misses me a lot [this is externalization plus disavowal because what she means by this wording is "I do not miss her"]. And I wonder if it's because the minute she's not there, if I've gotta kind of make her unreal [a defensive derealization to ward off pining after the hometown girl friend and, symbolically, home]. I put her in a timeless slot and I expect her to stay the same and, you know, like I can take her out of a drawer [a defensive facilitation of the illusion of having control over the presence or absence of another person].

T: Yes.

P: But it's the same with my family. I don't get homesick [disavowal of inhibited ideas; she does not acknowledge or experience potential emotions such as longing].

T: Yes.

P: I hardly ever get, every once in a while [we infer the underlying thought to be she "hardly ever gets homesick," followed by a softening of her statement "She gets homesick every once in a while," a switch from disavowing to proclaiming the experience while minimizing it. By the phrase once in a while she means **only** once in a while. She also leaves the other person in the communication with an indefinite topic and little to say except "yes" or "what?"].

In these statements, there is an indication of both central conflicts and habitual defensive strategies. She struggled between needs for dependence and independence. She wanted to think well of herself but tended to be self-critical. She wanted others to like her, yet criticized them. She wanted to be different from her mother yet felt a pull to identify with her or yield to her. She wanted to forget her mother's rebukes but could not put them out of mind.

Diagnosis from an Information-Processing Point of View

What do these ideational and emotional conflicts and her habitual styles of avoidance mean in terms of traditional diagnostic considerations? Her conflicts and defensive styles are sufficiently general to remove her from being classified as any particular personality type. Like the histrionic personality, she used repression and denial to avoid anxiety and guilt over attachment and separation issues. In interpersonal behavior she was dramatic in order to gain attention. Like the compulsive personality, she used intellectualization, undoing, role reversal, and isolation to avoid strong feelings, especially in power struggles, where there was the threat of being either too strong and dominant or too weak and subordinate. She engaged in power struggles but feared the resulting victory or defeat. When she got something from a relationship, she was not sure she wanted it. Like the narcissistic character, she tended to slide meanings about from moment to moment through generalization, externalization, minimization, and disavowal. She also tended to externalize attributes that threatened deflation of her self-esteem, and to show off to get support and to stabilize her self-confidence.

Microanalysis by the Thematic Progression Format

By examination of multiple sections of the transcript it is possible to reconstruct the themes, emotional threats, and defenses into simplified constellations, following the format of Figure 10. The first example of such a reconstruction models ideas related to her depressed feelings. In Figure 11 separate facets of the suggested format are indicated in the left margin. All subsequent figures will use an identical format. Once the reader becomes familiar with this structure, the figures will be easier to read than they may at first appear.

A suggestion of the crude relationship of the modeled aspects of information processing to states and relevant images of self and other is also indicated, although states and role schemata are on a somewhat different level of abstraction.

Figure 11 can be read by beginning with the event column: the news that her brother is dead, the memory of the funeral, and of her mother asking her to stay at home. Her response to these occurrences was a desire to stay at home for good. This respondent idea was a regressive step, conflicting directly with her aim to become an independent adult. A match between the respondent idea and the strong wish to become independent was not possible; the sets of ideas are

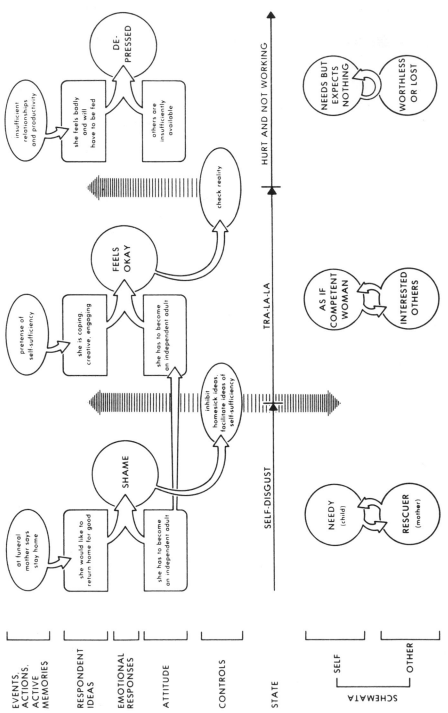

Figure 11. The Homesickness Constellation Leading to Depression.

discrepant. When ideas were actually processed, this incongruency led her to a feeling of shame. The threat of becoming ashamed motivated several control operations. In the model of Figure 11, one control is the inhibition of the idea of being homesick. Contrary ideas were facilitated, filling her awareness with thoughts about her own self-sufficiency. In addition, she kept the entire dependency–independency theme at a distance, did not allow herself to realize the degree to which she was caught up in it, and discounted it on any occasion, in evaluating its importance.

As indicated in Figure 11, the need to avoid self-disgust because of the threatening emergence of regressive dependency wishes led to controls that transformed her state. She pretended self-sufficiency and experienced her *tra-la-la* state. When she thought of herself as competent and on her own, there was a good match with her enduring attitude, the idea of becoming independent and mature. She responded to this good match by feeling good; she wished to stabilize herself in this pleasurable state. Unfortunately, she was unable to do so. Her behavior was not sufficiently effective to maintain her self esteem and she lacked sufficient levels of interpersonal attachments to sustain herself with support. Recognition of these reality situations made her again think of herself as weak, defective, and needy. Even when current reality did not trigger more negative self-concepts, the intrusive memories of her "bad behavior" at the funeral could do so.

The good feeling of thinking of herself as coping effectively, in accord with her strong aims to become independent, could not be maintained. Her relationships and personal productivity were not sufficient enough to sustain good images of herself. This led, as shown on the right of Figure 11, to respondent ideas of bad feelings about herself and her symbiotic need to be fed. When this concept was related to a shifting view of the relationship of herself to others, she felt depressed. That is, when she felt bad for these reasons, she also tended to shift to an enduring attitude in which the only others available to her were worthless, and worthwhile others had been lost. In ideational form, this role schema led to a concept that insufficient help was available, hence the depressive affect evoked by the mismatch between her desires for nurturing and the unavailability of supplies.

Again, this is reductionistic simplification, but it describes important interrelationships of ideas, feelings, and controls and prepares the way for an analysis of the process of therapy as related to specific themes. It also indicates the important ideational meanings and emotional responses that relate to the core images or schemata of self and others.

Another constellation of ideas, emotions, and controls concerns the memory of her behavior at the time of the funeral when she conducted herself in a silly and joking manner, did not cry as much as others would think proper, and was accused by her mother of being silly. This theme, modeled in the same format, illustrates her tendency to feel guilt and anger, and her use of both externalization and role reversal to avoid such feelings. The respondent ideas to this memory were that behaving as she did meant she was selfish or at least very self-centered, and this conflicted with an attitude that the self should be less important or subordinated to others. Her mother had frequently told her that she felt good about the subordination of her own needs to those of her husband and children. Particularly, at the time of the brother's sudden death, the patient felt that she ought to care more about what had happened to her brother than she did about herself, to be selfless rather than selfish.

The comparison of meanings between the idea that she was selfish and the moral injunction to be selfless tended to evoke guilt. She used externalization to avoid a sense of guilt or shame, feelings she believed would be painful and intolerable. She accomplished this defense by inhibiting from representation the ideas of herself as silly, and not crying. She also facilitated representation of contrasting ideas. One set was that her mother was bad. That is, she observed that her mother not only wept "authentically" but **used** weeping to get attention. In this way she could see her mother, rather than herself, as the one who wanted attention. Another set of contrasting ideas was simply that she was sad, but that her sadness was so strong that she **had** to bottle it up, and that made **her** the saddest of all.

As shown on the right side of Figure 12, labeling mother as the selfish one was motivated by defensive aims. This view was supported by a memory of how, at the funeral, mother received a great deal of sympathy for her grief. This view of mother was then matched with the attitude that a person should be selfless. The incongruence led her to view her mother with contempt and anger. Such emotions blunted her tendencies to feel ashamed or guilty about her self-centeredness.

Contempt and anger for her mother was also dangerous. She was vulnerable to feeling anxious or guilty about the degree of rage she could experience toward her mother. This danger could be thwarted by another role reversal. She could again see herself as bad or wrong. That is, she could oscillate back and forth in continual undoing, not feeling either guilt or anger to a degree that would be associated with any strong emotional experience. Intellectualization and generalization of ideas helped her escape further from the threat of these emotions.

Another ideational constellation is also relevant to the first part of Figure 12 in that it depicts her as doing wrong and leads to guilt. This constellation is the progressive version of the dependence–independence

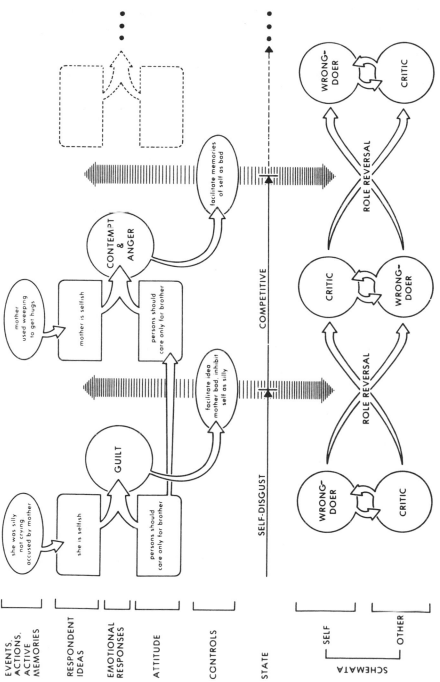

Figure 12. The Funeral Constellation Leading to Oscillation between Guilt and Anger.

conflict. The event, and active memory, was that at the funeral her mother asked her to return home to live. Her respondent ideas were that she wanted to continue her life away from home (to become independent), and that this would hurt her mother, who might also see it as selfish. From the viewpoint of the abiding attitude to not hurt one's mother, her decision to leave again would tend to evoke guilt. This is, then, the progressive version of the conflict shown as regressive in Figure 11. The emotion, control, and role relationship oscillations would proceed as indicated after guilt in Figure 12.

SUMMARY

The central ideational themes, conflicts, and unresolved problems for the time in question can be described in a way that shows the interaction of the patterning of external events with ideational flow, emotional response, control efforts, and the alteration of inner models. The thematic progression format can be used to show a typical evolution of ideas. This can begin with events or active memories of events that lead to respondent ideas. These respondent ideas are then examined as they interact with personal attitudes. Emotional reactions to this ideational comparison are depicted and are seen as instigators of controls that may alter the sequential flow of ideas and actions. One way controls are seen to operate is by alteration of the representation of ideas and feelings. Another way is by alteration of those self-concepts and role relationship models that are dominant organizers for a given state of mind. In following this evolution, one describes habitual defenses and conflicts as well as currently important problems and unfinished business.

By this point, then, one has stated what one can about the problems and recurrent states of the person, added inferences about schemata, and described the kind of problems under consideration as well as the form of decision making. These summaries will have included the intrapsychic and psychosocial dimensions. Even biological dimensions are included, as when such impairments of information-processing capacity are described. We are now ready to examine the processes of change by a review of these same facets.

II

Processes of Change

Analysis of a situation that changes requires description of a baseline from which to measure that change. That baseline has already been established by describing the pertinent patterns of the prechange level of the patient in terms of states, schemata, and information processing such as conflicted emotional themes and styles of control. Shifts from this baseline can now be analyzed to determine where, how, when, and why they occurred.

When the key to change is a therapy, the analysis of the process is complicated by the presence of the therapist, another person who will have his or her own states, roles, and styles of information processing. From the standpoint of logic, one should have described these salient patterns of the therapist at the baseline or pretherapy period. But for expediency, qualities of the therapist will be incorporated into the ensuing discussion of methods for analyzing the change process.

The interrelation of change, processes of change, and therapeutic technique is an area that has not yet been fully illuminated by scientific inquiry. Yet, to my knowledge, there is no other area where the interaction between what is observed and theory about what will be observed is more tightly meshed. Because of this, it is necessary to present not only a method for studying and describing change but a theory of how and why change takes place in psychotherapy. Because others may approach such clinical data with different theories, and therefore make other observations, I plan to present as much direct clinical material as possible without overburdening the reader. More extensive excerpts from transcripts of the 12 treatment hours are added as a supplementary resource in appendices. Since the main areas of complexity between theory and observation lie in the analysis of relationships and the examination of modifications in the processing of information, excerpts from the therapy were extracted twice, once from each point of view. The reader may choose to read these appendices after completing the text or to read the section on relationship after reading Chapter 6 and the section on the processing of information after reading Chapter 7.

CHAPTER FIVE

Modification of the Transition between States

Step 5. State: *Review entry into and exit from the states listed in Step 2 as they occur in therapy or are reported for current outside-of-session relationships. Divide the therapy or time of change into phases according to times of transition in state patterns, such as changes in typical state occurrences or cycles. When indicated, describe the states of the therapist or therapist and patient as a pair or small group. Describe the effect of interventions on the transitions between states. Include the effect of new external events on states and continuation of process after therapy when such data are available. If medication has been used, describe changes in states in relation to the time of use of the pharmaceutical agents. Include description of economic, environmental, or social situational changes.*

The crudest levels of change in problematic states, such as those of anxiety or depression, will be the first to draw the observer's attention. One can proceed gradually from there. In looking for changes in states, one attends to (1) differences in the quality of states already described, (2) altered frequency or duration of these states, (3) new states, and (4) changes in the conditions that evoke transitions from one state to another. Once preliminary patterns of state change have been identified, it may then be possible to define phases of therapy in terms of the frequency and quality of states.

When gross patterns of change in state have been clarified, one can go back over the data to see how interventions affect the state qualities or state transitions of the patient. This is equivalent to the cycle of states as described in Chapter 2, and that precursor will prove valuable at this stage. Interventions as illustrated here are the communicative acts of the therapist, but the events of the outside world may be included in the analysis, as may physical events such as prescription of medications, relaxation techniques, or exercises. For example, if the patient is given antianxiety or antidepressive medication, it will be important to compare for change in states and state transitions before and after that intervention, just as the effects of interpretation, confrontation, or advice may be examined in terms of the same changes and transitions.

ILLUSTRATION

The cycle of states depicted for Janice in Chapter 2 is reproduced here for convenience (Figure 13). The main states during the therapy hours were *tra-la-la* and *hurt but working*. The *competitive-critical, hurt and not working, crying,* and *acute self-disgust* states emerged clearly but were momentary in duration. The relative frequency of states, especially *tra-la-la* and *hurt but working,* marked off phases of the treatment.

During the 12 hours, the therapist appeared to be in four main states. In one he was inactive, somewhat cool and watchful, with occasional momentary and inhibited expressions of disinterest, frustration, irritation, or skepticism. This usually occurred when Janice remained in the *tra-la-la* state for an extended period of time. She seemed alert to this and occasionally responded with less pretense. At other times the therapist was active, more warmly engaging, and mildly hopeful in manner. During such periods, he often organized and structured preceding information about her past or current life choices. This state usually occurred when Janice was in the *hurt but working* state but, by the midpoint of therapy, proved especially effective in deflecting her from a nonproductive *hurt and not working* state.

In his third state, the therapist was verbally inactive but nonverbally kind and in close contact. This tended to relate to Janice's *hurt but working* and also her competitive state. The fourth and final state of the therapist was less frequent but quite noticeable. He was active, earnest, leaning toward her, and pressing her with statements or with a focus for her attention. This occurred most noticeably after she had been in the *tra-la-la* state for some time, and would cause a transition to the *hurt but working* state. The therapist also would enter this active state when Janice executed a seemingly successful defensive maneuver and was in transit from the *hurt but working* to the *tra-la-la* state, and was often successful in deflecting her from this state.

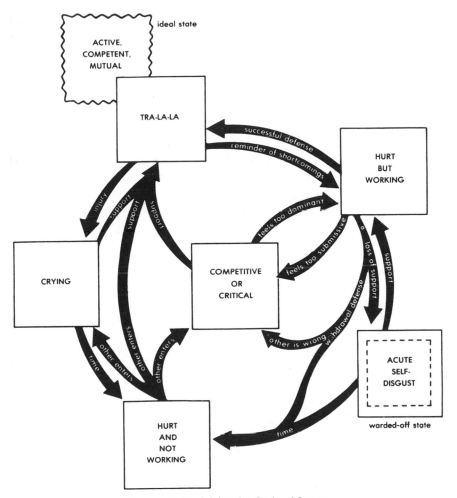

Figure 13. Model for the Cycle of States

The experiences of patient and therapist as one joint entity in this therapy could be called **monologues, dialogues, tests,** and **silences**. When **monologues** occurred, it was almost always the patient who talked and the therapist who listened. **Dialogue** afforded an exchange of communication. During this exchange, however, the therapist rarely spoke more than three sentences in a row, and usually uttered single phrases, directed toward clarification, accentuation, or focusing of attention. **Tests** were mild verbal assaults or ploys essayed by either person. These will be illustrated in Chapters 6 and 7. **Silences** were episodic, lasted only a minute or so, and ended easily.

There were five phases delineated by the states of the patient and the therapist and their experience as an entity. They can be described briefly and in order.

Phase One occupied the first two hours. During this time, Janice was mostly in the *tra-la-la* state; she tested herself in this situation and she tested the therapist to determine the range and variety of his responses.

Phase Two, which occupied hours 3 and 4 found her more turbulent. The *hurt and not working* state emerged more clearly as both Janice and the therapist revised errors made during tentative therapeutic agreements in the first two hours, especially those concerning the focus as mourning her brother's death.

Phase Three occupied hours 5, 6, and part of 7. There were transitions between the *tra-la-la* and *hurt but working* states as she tested the therapist and the growing relationship between them to see if he would dominate her and force her to identify with his values. These struggles centered on attempts by the therapist to encourage confrontation with her frustration concerning her aims to become independent from her family, and expression of this frustration.

Phase Four covered part of hour 7 and hours 8, 9, 10, and 11. During this phase there was transition between *tra-la-la* and *hurt but working* states, but there was less "hurt" in the latter state, and the main working through on separation versus dependency and identification themes, the working through of bad self-images, and these issues as they related to the funeral and visit home occurred. In addition, the issue of separation from the therapy was present here, but not as prominently as in some brief therapies. Janice began to experience sadness about the loss of her brother during this phase.

Phase Five was simply the last hour, when she was somewhat more detached from the therapist, and generally reviewed the main themes of the therapy.

Effect of Therapist Interventions on Changes in State

The long-range aim of the therapist was to help her achieve the ideal state of being and feeling like a competent woman. The short-term goal was to help her to work in therapy. This meant that the therapist had to aid her in leaving the *tra-la-la* or pretending state. When she was warding off conflict in this state, he confronted her by attempting to focus their joint attention on her current problems. This sometimes effected a transition into a *working* state where she examined her short-comings. Once she was in a *working* state, he tried to stabilize it by reducing injuries to her self-esteem, and thus preventing transitions to either *self-disgust*, or *hurt and not working* states. He countered the defenses and evasions that led her back to a *tra-la-la* state and dealt with her role reversal attempts in an effort to prevent transition to the *competitive* state.

With these efforts on the part of both patient and therapist during the 12-hour therapy, there was increased time spent in *working* states as compared to the *tra-la-la* state. This main change in the quality and frequency of states occurred in hours 8 through 11 and was associated with the establishment of the therapeutic alliance, described in the next chapter. Also, as already mentioned, there was a modification of the *hurt but working* state where she came to feel less hurt. There were fewer troubled facial expressions and more persistence in collaborative efforts to understand what was happening. She could confront increasingly threatening information about herself. She never became too comfortable in the *working* state because, in effect, the ante was always raised. She brought up warded-off contents whenever the situation became safe (Weiss, 1967). As therapy progressed, she was able to describe herself as spending less time in the *hurt and not working* state outside of therapy. Her behavior at work stabilized after the fifth hour or so and led to a major reduction in the threat of job loss.

SUMMARY

The first approach to describing change is to look for shifting patterns of state frequency, state quality, and state transition. The states of the therapist, or therapy dyad, may be an added component of state analysis. Gross patterns of state changes can be delineated as phases of a change process. The effect of interventions on states, especially as they influence state transitions, will be an important aspect of this stage of analysis.

CHAPTER SIX

Development of Views of Self and Interpersonal Relationship Patterns

Step 6. Relationships: *For each phase of therapy described in Step 5 describe changes in interpersonal relationships and self-concepts. Use the labels for self and other roles defined in Step 3. Discuss separations and new attachments. Then discuss the various relationships of the patient with the therapist, including social alliances, therapeutic alliances, transferences, and countertransferences. Indicate dilemmas of the therapist caused by alternative relationship views by the patient. The sequence of tests by the patient for relationship potentials, and the therapist's manner of dealing with these issues, can be summarized. Discuss actual and potential errors of technique provoked by the patient or made by the therapist. Describe useful and unhelpful techniques for dealing with relationship issues.*

During a period of change, as in psychotherapy, a person may work to alter his interpersonal behavioral patterns and the schemata by which they are organized, his self-concept, and his inner models of relationship. The changes that result can be simple shifts among existent elements in the repertoire of person schemata. **The usually dominant self-concept can be changed when another preexistent self-concept becomes predominant. This will result in state changes but not structural personality change. More important changes are those that further develop schemata, or that integrate dissociated ones into supraordinate forms.** These changes may include syntheses of previously incompatible models, or new versions of relationships with others.

The patient and the therapist each come to the therapy with their individual repertoires of role relationship models. As they interact they may develop new ways of relating. The patient learns from these new interactions by identification with the adaptive behavior styles of the therapist, and by unlearning maladaptive models. The patient learns by review of old patterns of interaction and by planning future self-images and roles. Naturally, the patient is also engaged in, and learning from, new interactions outside of therapy. This phase of discussion covers relevant patterns of change in self-images and role relationships.

BACKGROUND

The therapeutic relationship is the most thoroughly studied aspect of change in psychotherapy (Frank, 1974; Greenson, 1967; Langs, 1976; Gill, 1982a,b; Wallerstein, 1986). In the early part of this century, transference reactions were seen as a reenactment between the patient and the therapist of the patient's relationship with figures in his past life (Breuer and Freud, 1895/1957). Freud (1912/1958a) gradually distinguished between the variety of relationships that emerged in such roles. There were friendly, conscious, positive transferences; eroticized and unconscious positive transferences; and both conscious and unconscious negative transferences.

As recently reviewed by Langs (1976), the variety of transferences can be distinguished from the variety of real, therapeutic, or working alliances. Therapeutic alliances are special formations that differ from ordinary social relationships. In addition, the therapist has a variety of attachments to the patient, including his work and social roles and his potential transferences and countertransferences.

In considering these themes, Loewald (1960) has emphasized the special qualities of a transmutative therapeutic situation. **This opportunity for important changes occurs when the patient and the therapist consciously review simultaneous alternatives. They contemplate and compare roles of transference reaction with roles of therapeutic alliance. There can then be a pivotal moment; primitive schemata can be revised and new levels of mutuality attempted.**

Perhaps, paradoxically, it is because there is so much written about the therapeutic alliance and transference reactions (I mentioned only some major reviews) that one finds little in the way of a systematic approach for description of these processes when reviewing change. The matter appears complex, and a novice may not know where to begin. That is why, although many other approaches may be useful, a single, straightforward one is advanced here.

METHOD

One can begin by reviewing the change period in question and describing the **optimal relationship achieved by patient and therapist,** at whatever time in therapy it occurred. In what follows, this relationship is called the **therapeutic alliance** (Marmar, Marziali, Horowitz, and Weiss, in press). One can use it as a point of reference and then describe patterns that deflect from it. They will include attempts by the patient that fall short of a therapeutic alliance, as when, for security reasons (Sullivan, 1953), the patient tries to set up a **social** rather than a **therapeutic alliance.** Among other patterns of departure from the therapeutic alliance will be exploration of **transference** and **countertransference** relationship patterns. In these descriptions, the major movements and moments in the therapy, and the major entries, exits, and changes that involve other figures, will be included.

Therapeutic Alliance

It is important to start with an examination of the specific qualities of the therapeutic alliance because it differs so greatly for each patient and therapist. The therapeutic alliance should not be equated with the ground rules of therapy, although efforts to stay within them will affect the establishment of the alliance. For example, a hypnotic treatment will of necessity involve an alliance different from that of a behavior therapy or a brief psychoanalytic treatment.

Even within a given type of therapy each patient and therapist will set up a specific alliance or several alliances. Such alliances will partake of the basic role relationship models available to the patient and will be closer in quality to one than it is to another in the patient's repertoire. Other role relationship models in the repertoire will, in turn, be found as the underlying organizations of transference patterns. Everything said here for the patient can also be said for the therapist.

There are often two trials that fall short or go beyond the establishment of a therapeutic alliance. One tendency involves the patient seeking to elude a relationship in which an encounter with his difficulties is unavoidable. He tries instead to establish his most adaptive social relationship, presenting a facade of normality to the therapist. The second tendency is toward transference. The patient not only enters into the therapeutic alliance but is tempted to go beyond it into a zone where the therapist is used for gratification or for restoration of lost ties to another person. This view of change processes in terms of relationships is presented in Figure 14.

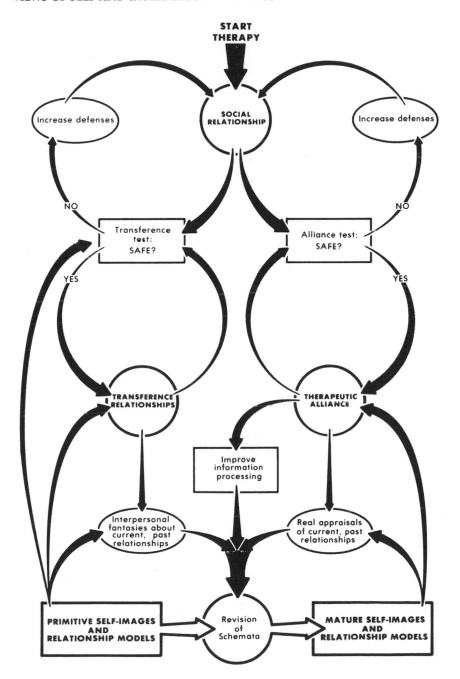

Figure 14. Development and Change in Role Relationship Models during Therapy.

Tests

The patient checks the therapist for responsivity, and himself for safety of responsivity. He tests the situation to see if a social interchange will be enough, to see if the match is stable enough to warrant a therapeutic alliance, and he tests it for transference potentials (Langs, 1976). These transference tests are to determine not only what wishes might be gratified but what fears are warranted. In a way, the patient does not want genuine transference-gratification because he has been troubled in his real life by repetition of such relationship gambits. He wants to see that the therapist will not allow a transference relationship to be acted through rather than worked through. The tests for transference potential, if handled well by the therapist, will strengthen the therapeutic alliance (Langs, 1976; Weiss, 1967; Weiss *et al.*, 1977; Weiss and Sampson, 1986).

There is another common variety of test, one of role reversal. The patient places the therapist in his most difficult role or dilemma and then watches to see how the therapist will handle it. The ability to handle it is then copied by the patient, and seen by him as a reason or validation of the importance and the benefits of the therapeutic alliance. Identification of these various tests for social, therapeutic, transference, and role reversal possibilities will be used as steps built upon the role relationship models outlined earlier for the specific patient and will further clarify each step.

The above statements seem to assume that a therapeutic alliance develops, that transference comes mainly from the patient, and that change is for the better. But a therapy can be analyzed in this way even when the therapist has introduced distortions, when there has been acting out of complementary transference and countertransference reactions, when the patient has identified with bad qualities of the therapist, and when a negative therapeutic reaction has occurred. For example, a misalliance may have been the prominent feature in a stalemated therapy or one that ended poorly. The first step would be description of this misalliance, its basis in the relationship schemata of the patient, the therapist's efforts or failure to correct it, and the course of deterioration over time.

Such patterns can be checked by taking short segments of therapy and applying microanalytic methods. These methods expand upon the verbal statements by adding inferences about what was meant and what possible reactions might follow the particular communication (Labov and Fanshel, 1977). If the described relationship patterns of the change process have explanatory power, then they will match well with the moments of action and reaction described in the microanalyzed segment.

A useful method for such microanalysis is the listing of communications by message units in a tabular fashion. Then the essential message can be restated, with addition of various possible meanings to each message. For each possible meaning, one or several reactions by the other person can be cited. The role relationship of the action and reaction can then be added to the table. This will be illustrated in what follows.

Microanalysis can continue endlessly, and its fundamental purpose must be kept in mind to avoid unnecessary preoccupation. In examining change one looks for pivotal moments, when the person could repeat a familiar but maladaptive pattern or select a less familiar, more adaptive pattern. In therapy these pivotal moments often occur when the patient interprets a message from the therapist according to the therapeutic relationship, the transference relationship, or a social relationship. Detailed analysis of any one of many such moments in therapy may clarify the repetitive transactions that facilitate change. This will be as important when change is negative as when it is for the better.

As mentioned earlier, events about relationships outside the therapy should be included in this phase of configurational analysis. As with events in the relationship with the therapist, happenings and behavioral pattern shifts should be related to the inner models of the patient. The difficult task will be, as with the therapist–patient relationship, determining where there is a movement in terms of altered dominance of existing models, and where there is a structural change in the models themselves. Such structural change may include new models, recombination or integration of models, and softening of some qualities of a given model.

Illustration

The Therapeutic Alliance. For Janice the therapeutic alliance corresponded most closely to the role relationship in which she was learning and needing to learn, and the other, the therapist, was a teacher strong enough to help her. While working on a basis for the therapeutic alliance, (a) she viewed herself as a person "en route" to maturation into adulthood although at present impaired by immature attributes; (b) she believed the therapist viewed her that way; and (c) the therapist **did** view her in that way. Reciprocally, (a) the therapist viewed himself as a calm, psychologically knowledgeable, hopeful, interested, and persistent teacher; (b) the therapist believed the patient viewed him that way; and (c) the patient **did** view him in that way. Without stating it crudely as "mature or immature," the strength of the alliance rests on such reflections and on the shared role concepts of the patient and therapist.

In this alliance Janice was able to see herself as giving information about her impairments. In a complementary fashion she saw the therapist as seeking that information by efforts toward increasing her awareness, by clarifications, and by interpretive constructions of meaning. She saw him as a teacher who benignly probed for weaknesses in order to help her to gain strength. She also saw him as interested in his role, and as interested in psychological knowledge and the process of imparting it. He worked on her behalf, but he also stood for fidelity to reality. He was not going to take on responsibility for her total care or welfare.

She could identify with his stance and join in it; she too was seeking information about her impairments and knowledge of how to change. Within their different and complementary roles, they worked together for change, could take pleasure in progress, were gratified when a goal was approached or a resistance or struggle worked through.

Within this alliance the therapist was able to see through her pretenses, could tactfully point out lapses from the role of a learning student, and tolerated her competitive struggles. It was important for Janice to see herself as an intellectually alert student, a person in control of the learning process, and one not overwhelmed by recognition of her impairment of underdevelopment. Both felt she was able to face the tasks of self-confrontation in the therapy and that responsibility for her life decisions resided with her.

As indicated in the previous section on phases, this alliance developed very slowly over the first 6 hours, but seemed to be fully established by the end of hour 7, allowing working through of important conceptual constellations during hours 8 through 11. The 12th and last hour was a review, with detachment from the therapeutic relationship and resumption of a social relationship.

During the first half of the therapy, before firm establishment of the therapeutic alliance, instability of role relationship was noted. The common shifts between relationship models were those already described in Chapter 3 and the relevant figure is reproduced here as Figure 15. As indicated in the figure, a ploy for resisting the **therapeutic alliance** was to see herself and the therapist as intellectually engaged, interested, and competent, as in this kind of social relationship. For her, this was a pretense; she came to therapy motivated to receive help for her impairments. Confrontation with these aims caused transitions from the *tra-la-la* to the *hurt but working* state. In other words, confrontations led from the pretense of being competent to reexperienced awareness of self as having limitations. As she developed the student–teacher alliance, she came to find the role of being "yet a learner of adult life" more acceptable. As this became easier there was less potential for hurt and shame, and

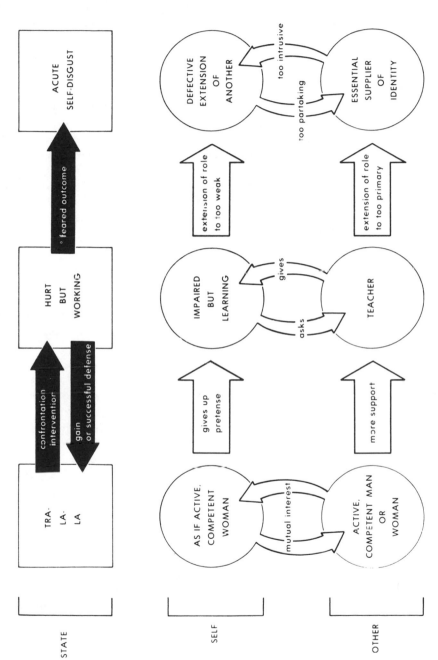

Figure 15. A Format for Modeling Role Relationship Characteristics of Common State Transitions.

so less need to escape from the working state and its self-images as a learner, back into the *tra-la-la* state with its "already competent" self-images.

Tests. One tendency to misalliance, then, was to present herself as too well, as already a competent woman, and to set up the **social relationship** of intellectual companions. This was, after all, the stance she took with friends and at work. These presentations also functioned as tests to see if the therapist could be taken in or if he would insist on therapeutic work. It was a misalliance because the pretense was destructive; seeing herself as already competent interfered with her potential work of therapy.

There was another tendency to misalliance based on antithetical behavior (Langs, 1976). In that misalliance she would be seen as if she was doing very poorly and as if the therapist had to rescue her completely. Gambits toward such a misalliance were apparent early; there were repeated requests that the therapist agree to provide good images of her, that he dispel her depressions and stomachaches, and that he buffer her difficulties at work by giving her written excuses. These gambits occurred in the first 5 hours, were noted by the therapist, and were responded to in a way that strengthened the therapeutic alliance but avoided criticism of the testing attempts. This is illustrated in detail in transcripts in Appendix A.

Transferences. Tests for a possible misalliance also indicated a **potential positive transference**. If the therapist agreed to be a total rescuer, she could find in him an ideal parent (mother). This type of needy and weak self-image in relation to a totally rescuing other was expressed late in therapy in this way: "I wish I could get sick and be in the hospital, or go crazy and be in a mental hospital, or, you know, not have to be responsible." This **positive transference** potential was, however, antagonistic to the **therapeutic alliance**. Although it is called positive, because of some emotional aspects of attachment, it would bring her no pleasure or adaptive gain. She was troubled by her unconscious wish to regress to dependence on her mother or some other substitute. She had a stronger, more adaptive wish to become independent and she wanted to be independent without causing her mother to suffer as she broke away from her. Rather, she wished her mother to admire and love her for her adult self. In other words, it was important to this patient that the therapist neither seduce her to dependency nor allow her to only pretend to be independent, but that he side with her aims for eventual, competent, unisolated independence.

One of several **negative transference potentials** revolved around the same situation. If the therapist refused to provide supplies and rescue, she tended to feel frustrated, criticized, and defective. She then turned the tables, viewed him as bad or selfish, and criticized him. It was necessary to tactfully handle her critiques of his sexism and orthodoxy, in order to establish and maintain the student–teacher relationship. These alliance and misalliance configurations can be reconsidered by referring to Figures 15 and 16 presented in Chapter 3 (as Figures 6 and 7) and reproduced here. The therapeutic alliance is like the student–teacher state at the center of these two figures. The failure to set aside the facade of normality, one potential misalliance, is exemplified by the relationship of competent self to competent woman, shown as the basic relationship for the *tra-la-la* state in each figure.

As noted, the potential **positive transference** has a possible negative result, which is entry into the self-experience of being only a defective extension of another, a reason that contributes to her fear of entry into the **therapeutic alliance** (see Figure 15). To avoid this danger she tended to reverse roles, to avoid submission by struggles for dominance. Being in control would be good, but excessive dominance of the situation meant avoidance of painful topics, a stance contradictory to the **alliance**. The alliance was established by the therapist, who confronted her but did not force her, always showing that she had the choice and control over bringing forward information.

Another danger of a **positive transference**, of being supplied totally, was that she could slip toward her greedy, destructive self-image in relation to a depleted, cheated therapist. This would relate to the state of self-disgust and guilt shown in Figure 16. The specific concept behind this risk was that she would see herself as "bad" because she had taken advantage of the special interests of the clinic for stress response syndromes to receive unrelated therapy.

She tested the therapist to see if he would fulfill her **negative transference expectations**. In one potential **negative transference reaction** she would see the therapist as a superior critic in relation to herself as wrongdoer, as in Figure 17 reproduced here from Chapter 3 (where it appears as Figure 8). His role would correspond to a role her mother sometimes held, when criticizing her for being promiscuous, or a role held by father, who accused her of laziness. Such dangers would lead her to avoid expressing her troubled relationship with Phillip, her difficulties in working, or her reasons for coming into treatment. The therapist would only humiliate her if she admitted these concerns.

Initially, she felt she was **not** upset by the death of her brother and that she needed treatment because of recurrent depressions before that event. During the first phase of therapy she was afraid to present these reasons for wanting therapy because the therapist might then say that

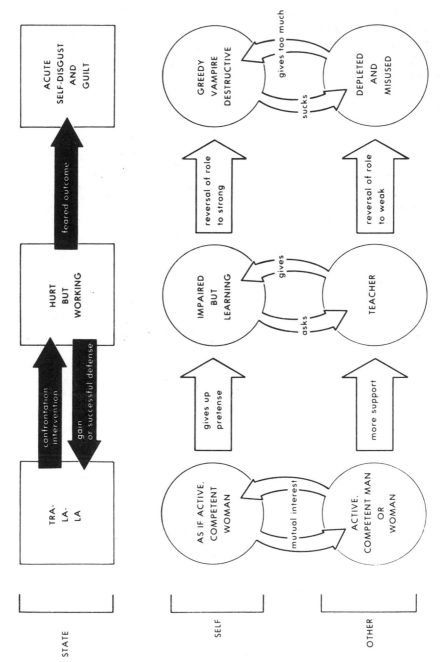

Figure 16. Main Role Relationships for the *Tra-la-la, Hurt but Working,* and *Acute Self-Disgust and Guilt* States.

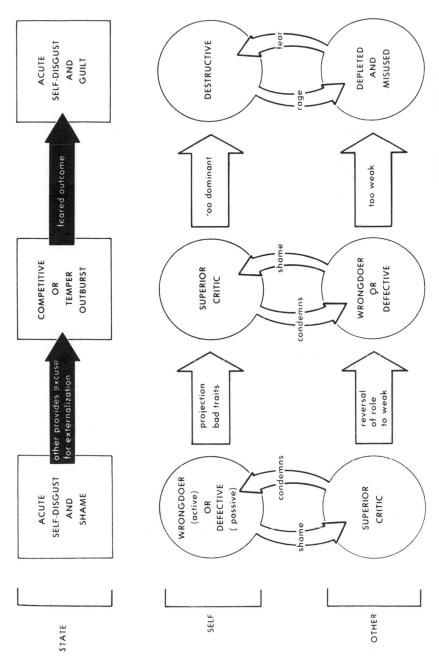

Figure 17. Role Relationships for the *Acute Self-Disgust and Shame, Competitive,* and *Acute Self-Disgust and Guilt* States.

she had come to the special stress clinic under false pretenses. The possibility for this **negative transference situation** was reduced and the alliance fostered when the therapist helped her to express these ideas while not criticizing her for "false pretenses" and not terminating her treatment as "inappropriate." Since he was also not going to allow her to procrastinate, or continue her treatment endlessly, she entered a zone where she could describe and examine negative self-attributes.

Because of her concern with not being seen as defective by an authoritative, rejecting person, her brother's death did serve as a ticket of admission to therapy. It was a clear insult of Fate, not her own fault or weakness. It attracted sympathy and could diffuse a focus on the developmental impairment that produced her depression. Here a partial **misalliance** stemmed from the above-mentioned therapist and clinic situation. The therapist and the clinic in which he worked were particularly receptive to her "stress event," the death of her brother. The matter was further complicated. She came in complaining of having suppressed her mourning over the death of her brother. Because of these factors a **misalliance** was established in the first interview, where the therapist tried to establish the working through of her grief responses to the brother's death as a focus.

He subsequently corrected this misalliance or error in focus, a correction that then fostered development of the **therapeutic alliance**. Otherwise, the therapist would have been seen much like her bad mother image: too intrusive and too self-preoccupied. Another **misalliance** would have been to then **exclude** the death theme. Correction was made in hour 7, to reinclude this theme, and that led to the working-through phase of hours 8 through 11 (also illustrated by transcripts in Appendix A).

Other elements of the therapy situation contributed to difficulties in establishing a **therapeutic alliance**. She was a research patient, and as such, the usual fee was waived. She gave consent to videotaping, audiotaping, rating scales, and teaching and scientific use of these materials. These factors limited confidentiality and also had a specific fit to her role relationship concepts. Her fear of humiliation, her interest in showing her good attributes, and her use of pretending as a defense were all heightened by the artifacts induced by recording the therapy. She had realistic fantasies of an eventual audience behind the therapist. She wondered how the therapist felt about being recorded and being onstage. He might be self-centered. In that way he could be seen as too much like her mother, who, she felt, manipulated her, so that she would be "Mother's own girl," and bolster Mother's image as "a good mother."

If he were like her mother, the therapist would want her to submit and to cry so that he could exploit her emotional display as a sign of his good technique, just as she believed her mother did, in fact, want her to cry "appropriately" at the funeral in order to demonstrate that her daughter, once "too hippy," now conformed to conventional behavior.

To recapitulate, a **therapeutic alliance** was gradually established, much like the relationship of a slightly wayward student to a tolerant but firm teacher. For her this was a progressive development. It led to unique experiences contrary to her current conflict with her mother. Her father was dogmatically critical but caring; her mother was also caring, but experienced as intrusive because Janice felt as if her mother imposed her own identity on her. She loved her parents, but she had to fight their injunctions to be like them and with them, and their criticisms or hurt feelings when she was unlike them or away from them. With the therapist she acknowledged her personal limitations without excessive self-criticism and confronted some of her own difficulties in making responsible decisions for her own life. In establishing this alliance, there was temporary stabilization of a real self-feeling, of "being on her way" but not yet "there," and so a greater tolerance for recognition of her personal difficulties.

The principal difficulty in establishing this relationship was her aversion to presenting information that made her appear impaired, and led to her habitual style of pretense. In the therapy, this manifested itself as pretending to be happy and satisfied, as resisting by attempting to establish an intellectual–social relationship, and avoiding a therapeutic focus. A single brief excerpt is presented here to illustrate the varied role relationship potentials in even a very brief therapy interchange.

An Example of Microanalysis of Relationships. Once the important configurations of role relationship are understood, small segments of the therapy can be "microanalyzed" using these patterns to organize the meanings in every fragment of communication. The explanatory power, the ability to understand communicative sequences, is one type of check on the validity of generalizations (Labov and Fanshel, 1977).

Microanalysis of the role relationships behind communications can be achieved with an almost random selection from the transcript of a therapy segment. One can quickly find a segment that seems intuitively to encapsulate repetitive patterns. In the following example, a section is selected from the third therapy hour, where the therapeutic focus is still at issue. Earlier in that hour the false-pretense issue and the potential misalliance of a focus on her grief over her brother's death were discussed. Janice brought up her "laziness" as a possible focus, a term by which she meant to label her lack of progress through current life tasks such as improving her work, interpersonal relationships, and personal skills. Here is the interchange that will be subjected to microanalysis.

P: [Coughing, sniff] Or . . . or, like saying, well, so I'm lazy. So what? So what's so bad about being lazy? You know, I mean, obviously I think there is something really, really **bad** about being lazy, but I'm trying to say, "OK, I'll let myself be lazy at times."

T: Oh, **there** is something you do experience. You experience yourself as being lazy sometimes.

P: Uh-huh.

T: It gets you into trouble and it **does** scare you.

P: Uh-huh. You mean that's a real feeling that I really know and I really have?

T: We could find out something about that because it's a real feeling that you really have, and there are real events, and you can place them.

P: Hm. I try to . . . to say, "Now this is not laziness. This is a need or I'm mad and I'm dealing with a problem, or something like that." But it all goes under the heading of laziness. And in some instances it is more excusable than in others. There are times when staying in bed and reading a book is okay. It's coping, or something like that, or recharging, or whatever. And there are times when it's just plain not okay, or if I've done enough coping.

     The statements can be examined in detail by dividing them into the literal statement, the essence of the communication, and interpretations of the various possible meanings of the remarks. These are the first three columns of Table 17. As shown therein, any communication, however short, has the possibility of multiple meanings. Each meaning or possible intention can provoke an even wider variety of responses. A selection of the most pertinent possible responses is included in the next column, "Possible Reactions." In the final column on the right side of Table 17, the role schemata as applied to that meaning and reaction are summarized, with an indication of the potential for **alliance, positive transference**, or **negative transference**. Note that each step in this segment of dialogue between patient and therapist is an oscillation between establishment and use of the **therapeutic alliance** and the role relationships of potential **positive or negative transference reactions** or failure to progress from social roles to a therapeutic alliance.

     Naturally, Table 17 oversimplifies; it selects only major roles. But it does list the multiple meanings and most typical "possible reactions" for this patient and this therapist at this time. The multiple meanings in the center of the chart are simultaneously present within Janice. She interprets the situation as being a **therapeutic alliance**, but at the same

Table 17. Microanalysis of Sequential Dialogue: Laziness Theme

Literal statements (from therapy hour 3)	Essential statements	Expansion of meanings	Possible reactions	Role relationships felt by patient — self	other
A. P: . . . or, like saying well, so, I'm lazy. So what? So what's so bad about being lazy? You know, I mean, obviously I think there is something really, really, **bad** about being lazy, but I'm trying to say, "OK, I'll let myself be lazy at times."	P: I am lazy.	P: She feels bad about being lazy.	T: Chooses laziness as focus	Therapeutic alliance — (Learner) ● — (Teacher)	
B. T: Oh, **there** is something you do experience. You experience yourself as being lazy sometimes. P: Uh-huh. T: It gets you into trouble and it **does** scare you.	T: You feel bad about acting lazy, and we can work on that.	1. T: Thinks she would like to get over being lazy. 2. T: Thinks laziness is one of her bad traits	1. P: Agrees to work on laziness, or explains why it is a mistaken focus 2. P: Refuses to agree on laziness	Therapeutic alliance — (Learner) — (Teacher) Negative transference — (Inferior wrongdoer) ● — (Superior critic)	

(Continued)

Table 17. (Continued)

Literal statements (from therapy hour 3)	Essential statements	Expansion of meanings	Possible reactions	Role relationships felt by patient — self	other
C. P: Uh-huh. You mean that's a real feeling that I really know and I really have?	P: Do you mean I feel lazy?	1. P: She does not offer to focus on laziness.	T: Repeats offer	● Therapeutic alliance	
			T: Interprets resistance or clarification of disagreement	Negative transference	
			P: Experiences interpretation as criticism; feels ashamed	(Inferior wrong-doer)	(Superior critic)
		2. P: Is not very lazy and therapist is criticizing her by thinking laziness is a problem	T: Insists she is lazy enough for it to be a bad trait		
			T: Backs off and apologizes for suggesting laziness is a problem	Negative transference, roles above reversed	
		3. P: Wants therapist to go on talking about laziness until he says something wrong	T: Goes on talking and says something wrong		
			P: Criticizes therapist	(Superior critic)	(Inferior wrong-doer)
		4. P: Wants the therapist to tell her more about laziness, to work for her, and to be interested in her	T: Is nice to her; explains and excuses her laziness, tells her how not to be or feel lazy	Positive transference	
				(Needy)	(Restorative rescuer)

D.	T: We could really find out something about that because it's a real feeling that you really have, and there are real events, and you can place them.	T: We can work on laziness.	T: Consider again if you want to work on your laziness.	P: Agrees to work on laziness, works on it
				P: Says why laziness is wrong focus, or she doesn't want to work on it
				P: Recognizes defensiveness ●

Therapeutic alliance

(Learner) (Teacher)

E.	P: Hum, I try to . . . to say, "Now this is not laziness. This is a need, or I'm mad and I'm dealing with a problem, or something like that." But it all goes under the heading of laziness. . .	P: I want to say I am not lazy.	P: Is ashamed of laziness and would like to avoid focusing on it	P: Goes on working on it
				P: Withdraws from working on it ●

Social relationship

(Interested adult) (Interested adult)

F.	and in some instances it is more excusable than in others. There are times when staying in bed and reading a book is okay. I'm coping, or something like that, or recharging, or whatever . . .	P: I'm not always lazy or very lazy.	P: Let's not regard laziness as a serious problem.	P or T: Withdraws from topic
				P: Contemplates topic further. ●

G.	and there are times when it's just plain not okay, or if I've done enough coping.	P: I am lazy.	P: Would like to work on this problem	T: Helps patient work on this problem ●

Therapeutic alliance

(Learner) (Teacher)

● = Reaction Selected by Respondent.

time she processes the communication in terms of the role relationships of social patterns or positive and negative transferences.

Multiple response possibilities are listed for each transition. The dark circle indicates the main choice of the moment; the other possibilities are not totally excluded, they are present but secondary.

This microanalytic approach shows how choice of wording conveys a great deal of meaning. One example is found in her use of the word "laziness." Her selection of this word sets up a situation in which the self-criticism that she has internalized from transactions with her parents can be reenacted socially. She regards laziness as a criticism that comes from outside; her father calls her lazy and stupid when he disapproves of her behavior, such as lying around the house. She does not feel lazy as much as she feels stymied in developing her life interests and threatened by facing her dilemmas and choices. She calls herself lazy in her fantasies. By offering the word "lazy," which the therapist then uses, she puts the therapist in the role of the critical parent. But the therapeutic alliance provided sufficient support so that progress could be made despite his unknowing use of this word.

SUMMARY

The relationships during therapy, the entrances and exits, the interaction with the therapist as well as the altered behavior patterns with others, are examined during this phase of configurational analysis. The goal of the pattern description is estimation of processes of change in inner models of self and relationship roles.

The variables that are frequently important in such processes of change include the social, therapeutic, and transference relationship possibilities with the therapist; relationship potentials that will be directed and organized by the basic inner models of the patient and the therapist. As the actual relationship changes, through the course of various trials, the inner models may shift. Estimation of these change processes is the key issue at this point. Such changes are choices, often new choices, made at pivotal points when there are possible alternative reactions to situations. The analysis of how such decisions are made is the topic of the next chapter.

CHAPTER SEVEN

Working Through Ideas, Feelings, and Modifying Controls

Step 7. Information Processing: *Classify interventions by the therapist in relation to key themes and defensive resistances as outlined for constellations of ideas, emotions, and defenses. Describe the focus of attention and levels of interpretation used by the therapist. Focus on work (or failure to work) on the main themes and defensive styles described in Step 4, on explanations of the shifting state patterns in different phases of therapy described in Step 5, and on explanation of the processes of changing relationship patterns described in Step 6. Describe how therapist interventions affected the patient's control processes and explain changes in the patient's key attitudes, beliefs, and ability to plan or restrain intended actions.*

As persons process information about their lives, modification of controls is central to effecting change. Excessive controls avert clear recognition of choices; on the other hand, insufficient controls may result in emotional flooding so extensive that it interferes with rational choice. An ideal state of regulation would be one that permits adaptive decisions.

Chapter 4 delineated important controls used in the pretherapy period. Chapter 5 indicated the relevant shifts in state that were the results of modification in controls. Chapter 6 indicated shifts in which role relationship models were used to organize interpersonal relationship patterns. These shifts were also caused by modifications of controls and the resulting choices. This step should focus explicitly on how and why controls are modified and how such modification affects the processing of problematic sets of information.

Modification of controls occurs as the internal or external situation is altered. There are many factors that can induce such modification. The correction of electrochemical imbalances will restore impaired capacities to full function and improve modulation of ideas. The same ends can be accomplished when insufficient support systems are corrected by improved family communication or by establishment of a therapeutic alliance. Habitually rigid control systems can be altered by suggestion or by training and practice in new ways of thinking and sensing. Unconscious control operations can be called to conscious attention and modified by volitional counterprocesses. The simple reduction of threats can make controls less necessary, just as promises of gratification can motivate control reduction.

Progression of thought occurs with the right kind of control modification. When emotional experience accompanies the progressive thought, it is commonly called working out or working through (Freud, 1914/1958b); Karush, 1967). This process includes increased clarity in assessing current problems, and leads to decision making. For example, reduction of stress can be achieved by either reappraisal of external threats or revision of internal models (Janis and Mann, 1977; Lazarus and Folkman, 1984; Horowitz, 1986). New decisions themselves alter the situation because they can reduce threat, which in turn allows some relaxation of the controls usually reserved for situations of danger. Immature models of reality can give way to development or shifts to more mature inner models. New conceptual and physical actions can be planned, tried, revised, and practiced. As these new modes of awareness, thought, expressions, and action become automatic, a modification of habitual forms of control occurs in a beneficial rather than in a vicious cycle.

BACKGROUND

As a result of work with his patient, Anna O., Breuer collaborated with Freud in describing the process of **catharsis** (Breuer and Freud, 1895/1957). To instigate this process, the therapist brought into focus the original moment when a symptom was formed, and then persisted in helping the patient to reproduce the ideas and feelings that occurred at that time. This intervention, sometimes associated with hypnosis, countered the inhibitory controls of the patient, who, in forming symptoms, both remembered and repressed certain aspects of inciting events. The aim of the intervention was to direct the discharge of impulses toward more adaptive objects by conscious choice rather than by the unconscious decisions that led to symptom formation. This is the essence of analysis of alteration in information processing. However, the explanatory theory proved too simplistic and later elaborations followed.

Freud experimented with interventions that might alter controls and lead to change. He moved from hypnosis to free association, a suggested mental set that led to conscious expression of warded-off ideas without the dominating role relationship implications of trance induction.

As a method for review of the change processes once they occurred, he suggested three subdivisions of ideas and feelings: conscious, preconscious (those accessible to consciousness), and unconscious (those that could not be consciously represented because of warding off). The process of change in the mind of a person was perceived as changing the status of various aspects of a thematic constellation. Associations with unconscious or warded-off information were brought to a conscious and hence more volitionally controlled level (Breuer and Freud, 1895/ 1957). One could divide a change period into phases, contrasting them according to the ideas that were conscious, preconscious, or unconscious during each phase, and explain transitions between phases by modifications in control (defense) and the interventions that led to these modifications.

These suggestions have proved viable in research approaches to studies of therapy process. Knapp (1974), Weiss and Sampson (1986), Sampson, Weiss, and Gassner (1977), and Blacker (1975) have distinguished phases of therapy and examined change as a result of interventions that led to the emergence of previously warded-off mental contents. Sampson and Weiss (1977), Weiss *et al.* (1986), and Caston (1977) have elaborated on the concept of warded-off mental contents, developing the theory of an unconscious plan. Analysis of change, according to the methods they suggest, includes description of the unconscious tests a patient may initiate to see if the therapist is for or against the plan, trials to see if the plan can safely become conscious, and eventual conscious recognition and deliberate action according to the plan.

Attention to the reordering of unconscious ideas is also seen as a useful way to review a process of changing sets of information by cognitive and behavioral theorists (Bower and Meichenbaum, 1984; Beck and Emery, 1985). Conditioned associations that are maladaptive and inappropriate are eliminated by techniques such as desensitization and cognitive restructuring (Lazarus, 1981). Preferential associations are established by operant conditioning using reinforcement (rewards) and deterrents. The process of conditioning can be analyzed in terms of altered response pathway probabilities, alteration based on transformation in the connection between associates or sets of information, and change in whether sets of information are expressed consciously or coded unconsciously.

METHOD

As mentioned above, analysis of change in the transformation of information begins with the selection of an important constellation of information, a selection already completed in Chapter 4. **Any alteration in this constellation during the change period is described in terms of the expression of warded-off ideas, new levels of awareness or differentiation of concepts, the sequential flow of the topic through various associations, decisions, changes in models, and the input of particular information that affected each transition.** This is a tall order and needs adjustment to each individual circumstance. But a key focus has been suggested: In order to describe, observe whatever input has affected the controls used by the patient to regulate the sequential flow of ideas and emotions.

In simplest form, here is one approach to the analysis of change in information processing. Take the constellation of information already described in Chapter 4. That description will have included provisional review of an ideal type of outcome (as originally detailed in Chapter 1) as a contrast to the pretherapy state. That is, the natural problem solving and completion properties of the mind for the particular discrepancy, incongruence, or conflict will already have been outlined. The controls or control failures that limit the person from reaching the ideal outcome will also have been examined. The state of irresolution as compared with the ideal problem-solving route will be anchor points for work during this step. Now the status of the initial constellation can be contrasted with its status during relevant phases of the change period. Observation and description should focus especially on input that appeared to affect controls and prevent solution of the problem. Modification of controls and the resulting flow of ideas and feelings toward decision and action will be central topics.

This focus on the input that influences controls includes attention to effects of the therapeutic relationship and transferences as discussed in Chapter 6, and differences in how information is processed in varied states as set forth in Chapter 5. It includes what the therapist suggests, tells, and teaches the patient to do as well as what behavior the therapist emulates. It includes patient behavior that is reinforced, responded to negatively, or ignored. Specifically, the effect of any particular technique should be discussed. For example, if the therapist used free association, dream interpretation, directed visual imagery, behavior schedules, role-playing, or techniques for thought-stopping, then the effects of these techniques in inducing or deterring change should be examined.

The effect of information from the therapist to the patient should be assessed. This includes the impact of advice, interpretations, clarifications, and confrontations as well as the effects of the patient's interpretation of other therapist actions such as prescribing or not prescribing medication, charging for missed hours, extending hours, empathically responding accurately or inaccurately, and so forth. The aim is to select the relevant actions, since any therapy is too rich in information to allow examination of all activity.

The selection of relevant variables may be determined, in part, by the type of therapy and its length. **In brief therapies, the focus may be more on working through a particular constellation of conflicted reactions and impulses. In long-term therapies, the focus may be on a modification of unconsciously operating defensive controls and decision making that revises more primitive self-images and roles in the direction of more mature representations.** The actions of the therapist, in any given phase of therapy, may also be assessed for depth and locus of attention. An example of levels and focus of interpretations is provided in Table 18.

When gross patterns have been abstracted, the validity of these patterns should be checked by finer-grained analyses. Microanalysis of process notes, or of transcribed excerpts of the therapy, is a useful method for checking validity. The large-scale patterns should allow relatively powerful explanations of immediate process sequences. The expansion of meanings from what is said to what is meant, and the various possible intentions beyond what is meant, is the essence of such microanalysis. These methods are better expressed in concrete illustration than by abstraction, since they must be flexibly altered to individual circumstances.

ILLUSTRATION

Previous levels of description have already clarified how Janice came for therapy when she felt depressed by the realization that her intended separation from home had not progressed as far as she wished. She came in a state of conflict intensified by both the death of her brother and her recent visit home for his funeral. She felt insufficiently competent and capable in her self-concept and insufficiently independent in her interpersonal behavior. Her wish for independence and her sense

Table 18. Levels of Interpretation[a]

	Content areas	Current situations	Therapy situation	Past
Link between external situation and personal responses {	1. Stressors and stress responses	Intentions of how to respond	Expectations of treatment	Relevant experience of previous stress events
	2. Pending coping choices and conscious scenarios	Conflicting aims of how to respond	Dilemma analysis of what to deal with first	Long-standing goals and habitual conundrums
	3. Avoiding of adaptive challenges	Threat and defense	Resistance to working through a conflicted issue	History of self-impairing character traits
	4. Repertoire of states of mind	Triggers to entry into problem states or exit from symptomatic states	States of therapeutic work and nonwork	Habitually problematic and desired states
Link between current problems and long-standing individualized personality patterns {	5. Expressed irrational beliefs	Differentiation of realistic from fantastic associations and appraisals		
	6. Repetitive maladaptive interpersonal behavior patterns	Interpersonal problems and self-judgments	Differences between social alliances, transferences, and therapeutic alliances	Abreaction or reconstruction of traumas and strains in relationship
	7. Self-concept repertoires and role relationship models	Views of self and others	Differences between social alliances, transferences, and therapeutic alliances	Development of role relationship models
	8. Warded-off unconscious scenarios and impulsive agendas	Urges, dreams, and creative products	"Transference neurosis"	Episodes of regression that uncovered warded-off aims in the past

Levels of analytical focus

[a]From Horowitz (1986b, p. 43).

of her own limitations in achieving it were reenacted in her actions and reactions to her mother during the funeral, at work, with her boyfriend, and with the therapist. She felt the need to break away from her current attachment to Phillip but could not do so because of anticipated loneliness. At work, she could neither accept direction from a supervisor nor carry out adequate independent work. In therapy, she presented a complaint (lack of mourning response) that she would not work on when urged to do so by the therapist. She was independent of him in this way but not so independent as to formulate by herself and work on a personally useful alternative theme. (For illustration of this point see the annotated excerpts of the therapy in Appendix B.)

The therapist gradually and repeatedly confronted her with this state of affairs, showing her how it affected immediate transaction as well as her other relationships. She faced these issues more directly after a series of preliminary tests to see if the therapist would insist upon making her submit to dependence upon him, in which case she would have to break away, or insist that she was already independent, and in that event would be lonely and despondent.

The ideal course of problem solving, at the most general level, would be for her to make plans and to act on decisions for her own self-development as an independent adult, and to explore her varied reactions to her brother's death. Her state of irresolution before therapy prevented her from thinking about her plans. Also, she was depressed, and would not confront her own reactions to her brother's death. Late in the therapy she was making plans for her self-development, and was experiencing some feelings of grief for the loss of her relationship with her brother. The intervening variables were her own natural tendencies toward these processes, facilitated by the relationship with the therapist, the opportunity for information processing of the therapy time, and the interventions of the therapist. Details of this overall statement will follow.

Working Through on the Homesickness Theme

The family reunion, a theme that related wishes and fears activated at the funeral to longer-standing problems of separation and independence from her mother, was called the homesickness theme in Chapter 4. At the funeral her mother asked her to remain at home and she had respondent wishes to do so that were incompatible with her stronger wish to become an independent adult. This contrast activated feelings of shame, a state of *self-disgust*, a role relationship as a needy child attached to a mother. She inhibited these ideas, disavowed and externalized them onto other persons, and pretended self-sufficiency. Figure 11

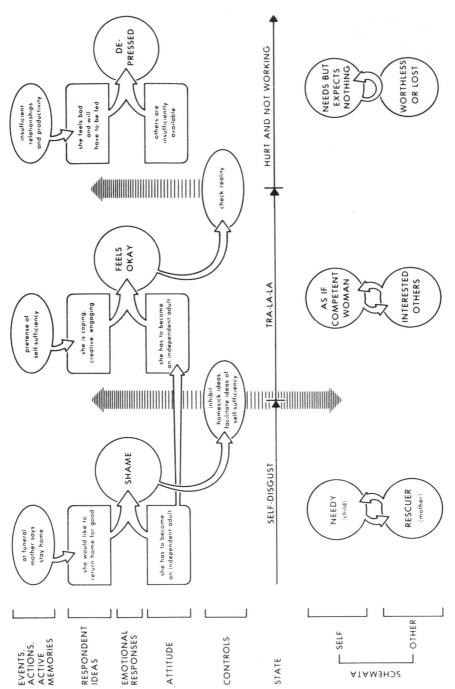

Figure 18A. The Homesickness Constellation Described in Step 4 as Leading to Depression.

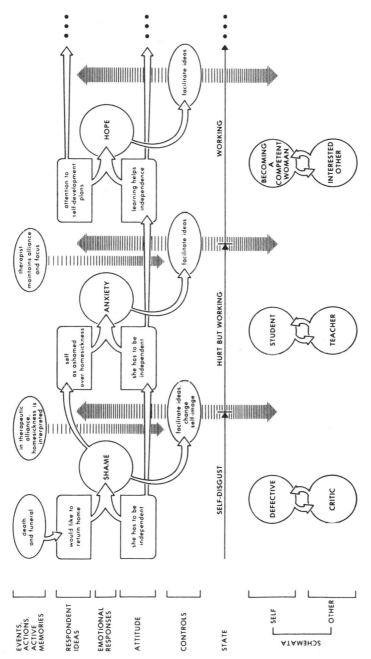

Figure 18B. The Homesickness Constellation Leading to Hope.

in Chapter 4 illustrates this constellation and is reproduced here as Figure 18A for convenient comparison to the therapy version, Figure 18B. The pertinent question for this step concerns changes in the status of this constellation **during therapy**, and an understanding of the input that instigated or facilitated these changes.

As already described, an indication of her initial defensive stance was found in the first therapy hour when she described a friend who missed her a lot, whom she did not miss. She added, "But it's the same with my family, I don't get homesick." When the therapist agreed with this, she hinted that it was not really the case by adding, "I hardly ever get (short pause) [homesick] every once in a while." This same defensive denial and reversal was present again in the second therapy hour when she said, "Did I tell you that I never get homesick? That I don't miss my family and I don't miss my friends?"

As a contrast, later in therapy she could acknowledge homesickness while maintaining her desire for independence. For example, in the 10th therapy hour she described how, on arriving home for the funeral, "I came off the plane with a lip-trembling kind of thing and at various times I could have fallen on her [the mother's] breast with tears and wailed." In the 11th therapy hour she was able to say, "When I think about it now, I think maybe that's what I wanted, you know, like you reach out and you loop each other's hands and you look into each other's eyes, and then you know something has passed between you."

The modification in acceptance of this theme was aided by the therapeutic relationship and, within that relationship, by clarification, confrontation, and interpretation. This process will now be illustrated in both macroanalytic and microanalytic detail.

On her own and early in therapy she could not stabilize a self-image as a student learning how to become independent, because she tended to be overly self-critical. She was threatened by the strength of her wish to return home and the associated self-image as a needy child searching for a rescuer. For these reasons she inhibited such ideas and facilitated counterideas of self-sufficiency (see Figure 18A). These controls impeded a planned approach to confronting and resolving her problems.

Effect of Therapist on Controls

Development and stabilization of the therapeutic alliance increased her tolerance for emotional responses. By his interventions the therapist gradually challenged her defenses and then helped her to process warded-off ideas. Put in slightly different words, within the therapeutic relationship the therapist could hold her to the homesickness versus independence theme by repetition, clarification, and interpretation. With increased tolerance for the anxiety it caused because of the safe relationship, she could pay attention to her conflict and plan on how to further her development. As she developed usable plans she felt increased hope and so could sustain additional facets of a working-through process. In contrast to the inhibition of ideas and pretense of self-sufficiency shown in Figure 18A, the effects of the relationship permitted the flow of ideas and emotional responses of Figure 18B, an overview of working through this theme.

Interventions by the therapist, as indicated macroanalytically in this figure, affected her controls. As it happened, these controls and the resulting defensive postures were dealt with in this therapy in an almost sequential order. The first issue involved interventions that counteracted her **inhibition**. Gradually, the therapist dealt with her switching between counterthemes. Then he intervened in relation to controls that accomplished defensive disavowal. In doing this, the therapist recognized the homesickness theme because of her defensive statements such as relatively gratuitous remarks about how she was not homesick. He was helped by a general theoretical understanding of the life cycle, and recognition that she had left home only some months prior to the death and the funeral.

Modification of Inhibition

In this first phase of treatment the therapist attempted to label warded-off ideas and feelings. One example of this type of clarification and interpretation in the working-through process is found in the fifth therapy hour. The therapist had used the word "lonely" to focus on an aspect of associations Janice had reported. She disagreed with the term but expressed a semblance of agreement about the feeling. He sided slightly with her disagreement but continued to confront her with the focus. Finally, he made a direct interpretation, saying that he thought she was homesick. She admitted it for the first time, but shifted from the *working* state to the *tra-la-la* state, going on to say it was not **people** she was homesick for, but her own childhood:

P: Uh-huh. Why would a [long pause]. It seems funny to say, lonely. I can't quite agree, but I can't disagree [pause]. In some ways, I had a really, really happy childhood.
T: Yeah. That's why it seems funny that I find myself using that word, yet you come across to me as being lonely.

P: Hm [pause].

T: I have a feeling that you're homesick.

P: Do you remember that hot weather? [pause] Um, what was it, a week and a half ago?

T: Yeah.

P: I got **so** homesick and that's the first time, really, since being out here. I've had one or two flashes. Once when it rained I thought of our house by the lake. I wanted to be there. But that hot weather [pause] in the summer its really hot and muggy, and [pause] I was really homesick, and it wasn't for the people, as they are now, it was for my childhood. I wanted to be at the lake. I wanted to go hiking with my brothers [pause]. You know, to fish [pause] sit in the living room and listen to the rocking chair creak, and somebody making tea, and **everything!**

T: Uh-huh. Well, it sounds nice.

P: Oh, it's really [pause] that's [pause] that's my home, by the lake.

Dealing with Switching Maneuvers

Another control that she used to deflect from processing ideas in this constellation involved **switching back and forth** between various attitudes. The therapist reacted to this with efforts to hold her to a specific attitude by imposing pointed questions and repeating frames of reference. Finally, he developed a specific nuance of technique, reinforced by Janice, who would then present her thoughts more openly. This nuance involved pointed reference to the defensive extremes of her switching pattern. His seizure of the disavowal pole seemed to prompt Janice to see the opposite position more clearly, and to state it more firmly, with less switching of attitudes, as if asserting her independence from his position. In doing so she often said more than she would have if the therapist had not seized the disavowal position.

An example is the following excerpt from the seventh hour. The therapist asked her to consciously intellectualize, to deliberately use a manner of control she ordinarily employed unconsciously.

T: But let's be, let's be very rational, very intellectual about it. What does it really mean to you that Sam is dead? In terms of you, what does it mean?

P: My life?

T: [Pause] What meanings does it have? Be very reasonable.

P: Well, nothing in [pause] in terms of the things like coming in and giving hugs and stuff. It's [pause] it means that occasional letter that isn't there, the admiration that he had for me. That asking for big sisterly advice kind of thing [long pause]. It means I don't like the mention of accidents [long pause]. Um, it doesn't mean [pause] doesn't mean anything that I can put my finger on.

T: Yeah. You know, we just look at that level, and **it doesn't have any big implications for your life on that level at all.**

(The therapist made his assertion at the disavowal position in her oscillation between "it does" and "it doesn't" have meanings. She then asserted the reverse of his statement more distinctly.)

P: In a way it does, because it [pause] it really brings home the reality of things. And, like, he was **there** [mumbles two words]. I hadn't seen him for a year, but I knew he was there. I had the faith; I believed he was there. And now he's **not** there, and I have to take **that** on faith too [sniffles]. I'm so, uh, what's real and what isn't? Is anybody real? Now, all these people that I remember, that I feel close to, that I have this faith in [pause] maybe they're not real either [pause].

T: Yeah. Well, it symbolizes, then, a larger realm of meanings which is that the family that you were attached to, your childhood and adolescent family, is no longer there for you. Because you're no longer a child or an adolescent. You've become independent [long pause].

Note that the therapist has again taken a position by saying that she has already become independent. He is saying, in effect, that she is not homesick. She can oppose him by saying that she gets homesick. She does this by saying, "When I get homesick," in what followed immediately after the above remark:

P: When I get homesick, I get homesick for childhood things and places. It's [pause] it's not a now [pause] a present-day homesickness. It's not like I physically need [pause] physically want to go back there and do what's going on now, or I'd live there now. I want to go back in time, too [long pause].

T: Sure. Then you had some pretty reliable ties with people. Your ties to Phillip aren't so reliable [pause].

P: No, not at all.

Counteracting Disavowal

While now in touch, at this phase of therapy (hour 7), with the conflictual constellation of ideas, she still maintained her distance from the theme by a failure to connect it with her needy child self-images and her use, instead, of competent self-images. In other words, she expressed the theme with objectivity rather than subjectivity, in the *tra-la-la* state rather than in a *working* state. The therapist's next task was to counteract the **inhibitions** by which she accomplished such defensive **isolation**. He confronted her with the treatment contract, focused on her as the subject of action, and repeated the issues without letting her get off the topic by either agreement or disagreement. Janice responded favorably to this maneuver and stabilized herself in the *working* state.

Here is an example from the ninth hour of how the therapist confronted Janice with distancing herself from a real encounter with herself:

T: I have a feeling you're moving away from me. I don't really have a clear picture of this at all, of where you stand on what you're doing and what you want to do. It just doesn't make enough sense to me somehow, which is why I feel you're not, not making it clear to me.

In a way, the therapist took her position. **He** was not clearly understanding her, just as **she** was not directly experiencing the theme. He repeated this challenge, asking that she make him understand. Because a therapeutic alliance had been established before this middle phase of therapy, he was able to be incisive. She shared his confidence in her ability to confront the warded-off ideas and feelings. Even in a struggle with him she could maintain a "strong" self-image to counteract the danger of emergence of her weak, dejected, and "disgusting" self-image. The excerpt continues with an example of such ongoing efforts at confrontation:

P: Well, it's 'cause it's not clear to me. You see, because I'm not thinking about what is this for, where am I going uh, what I'm doing is not working.
T: [Incisively] You're **not** working and you're **not** going to get married to Phillip and that's about where you're **at**. And . . .
P: [More argumentative] I'm waiting [pause] I'm waiting for Bob and Carol to come out.
T: Yeah, and they're bringing a fortune cookie with the answer to it in there?

This could be unnecessary sarcasm. However, the alliance is such that the patient understands the effort to use humor to perforate her rationalization for procrastinating.

P: [Subdued, earnest, reflective] Maybe. Yeah. They're bringing **me** [pause]. They're bringing [pause] a [pause] me [pause] that I like. They both **love** me.
T: Um-hm.
P: And they let me know it!

T: Yeah.
P: And they've known me for about ten years or more [pause]. And I'm counting on having their support and having them to bounce myself off of.
T: [Incisively] Yeah, but what about **me**? Why? Why am **I** in the dark now? Why am I feeling that I don't know what's going on with you?
P: I don't know. I don't feel that I'm trying to hide anything from you particularly.
T: MmHm.
P: It's probably just 'cause I don't [pause].
T: [Earnestly] I thought maybe you were sharing that feeling, though.
P: Like what? That I don't know what's going on?
T: Yeah.
P: [Somewhat petulantly] Well, I just don't want to **think** about it. I don't **want** to think, "Where am I going?" or What am I doing?"
T: [Firmly] Yeah, but what would you think of **me** if I let you get away with that?

This is an example of the therapist taking on her role; were he to let her get away with it, he would be the lazy one who allowed her life to stagnate. He is trying to help her to contemplate "laziness" by taking the role upon himself and asking her to react to him as lazy about understanding her.

P: No, I mean that probably why **you** feel hazy is because **I'm** being purposely hazy to myself.
T: [Firmly] Yeah, but what will you think of me if I don't say anything about that, if I just let it just roll on like that?
P: You've probably as fuzzy as I am.
T: We have a limited amount of time left. We have to finish by the end of the month. What if I just didn't, say anything, if I kept silent about that. I **mean** it. What would you think of me?
P: [Pause] I'm not say—[pause].
T: Would it be okay with you if I would not say anything else about that?
P: I might not even notice, probably, underneath. But, see, I'm not even sure what [pause] what it is that you're keeping silent about. And I [pause] I'm getting very confused, too.
T: MmHm. Oh.
P: [Very vague] Uhm, if you didn't think anything about your confusion, about where I am, and what I'm doing right now [pause].
T: Yeah, yeah. I guess one thing you'd be, it would be a version of laziness [pause] or whatever we're calling laziness, whatever. That's probably a pseudo-laziness [pause] whatever it is.

Here, the therapist joined in her vagueness. He, too, was fishing around, looking for the right leads, and letting her know that fishing around was "okay," not defective.

P: I don't know if that's what I am doing. It's [pause] fear and laziness. I don't
     want to think. I [pause] I want to kick the whole thing off. I don't want to
     [pause] I don't want to [pause] do much more than what I'm doing with
     you. I don't want to think about, uh [pause, then incisively] going to school,
     "Am I early enough?" I don't want to think about the fall. "Do I really want
     that job back again?" If not, what else? I don't want to think about the kind
     of person that I want to be.

The patient was being firm now, like the therapist, and may have
expected the therapist to sit back because she had been a good student,
saying something the teacher wanted to hear. But the therapist decided
to press on by having her contemplate how she would react to his taking
the "lazy" position.

T: Yeah, but the question says, "What will you think of **me** if **I** go **on** with
     that position?" I'll say, "Well, we only had a few more sessions, July, it's
     just a month. I don't want to [pause] I want to take [pause] I don't want
     to deal with her."
P: [Interrupts] I've got [pause] I mean [pause]—
T: [Overriding her] I don't want to deal with her. I don't want to deal with
     her in that way.
P: [Petulant] Um, I'd probably stop coming [pause]. If that was your attitude,
     I mean, if it came through to me that way, that you didn't **press** certain
     issues because "Well, we only have so much time and, after all, we can
     stick to the easy ones." 'Cause, uhm, that would make me feel [pause]
     rejected, and uhm, uninteresting, **unimportant**.

Repeated confrontation does not, with Janice, lead to some dramatic end-point of either revelation or decision. That is not her style. It
does, however, increase her time on the topic during the therapy hour.
More importantly, it increases her time on the topic outside of the interview, for it is her style to work over in her mind at other times the
incomplete, emphasized, or troublesome interchanges that occurred
during therapy.

Working Through a Troublesome Memory of the Funeral: Abreaction and Interpretative Reconstruction

The process of working through can be examined in somewhat
finer detail by reappraising the meaning of events at the recent funeral.
An important theme was an unresolved and unintegrated memory of
her silly or inappropriate behavior. At therapy onset, this theme was
warded off by inhibition and externalization, as diagrammed earlier in

Figure 12 in Chapter 4 and reproduced here as Figure 19A for convenient comparison. The relationship with the therapist and the focus on her own "bad" self-images allowed her to contemplate the meanings of this theme toward the end of the working-through phase of the therapy as is shown in Figure 19B. Instead of thinking in terms of accusations from another toward her, she was able to think of her self-accusations. Aided by the therapist, who focused her attention and made linking remarks, she considered the dynamics of the situation in relation to her struggles to separate from her mother and to keep from being like her.

Confrontation with the theme of her "selfish" behavior at the funeral made her feel guilty. The therapist, by means of interpretative reconstructions, helped her to go beyond these initial respondent ideas to more dynamic conceptualizations of the transactional situation. Within the therapeutic relationship the therapist encouraged abreaction, a detailed recollection, and attempt to relive in memory what happened at the funeral. This led to reorganized memories, and increased clarity in appraising her behavior. She saw that she had been motivated by such issues as fear of being like her mother and frustration at not getting more positive attention from her.

She recognized progress in understanding her motivations, and her sense of movement led to hope. Hope supported the working-through process. She could now acknowledge to herself that she had behaved "selfishly" at the funeral, but together with the therapist she knew that there were reasons for this behavior. She could identify with the therapist's attitudes that persons can have unconscious motives and do not have to be perfect to warrant attention. The match between these ideas, as shown in Figure 19B, led to remorse for her behavior, but remorse that was within tolerable limits. The result was a reduction in her potential for feeling guilty about this particular event. In a way this may have removed one block to examining the more extended meanings of her brother's death. Mourning for her brother was not completed during the therapy, but it did begin.

An Example of Microanalysis of Information Processing

Once the important aspects of information processing by the patient-therapist pair have been described, the explanatory power and validity of the expressed patterns can be checked by microanalysis of selections from video-recorded data. An apt sample for this process has already been stated: the section on page 126 from therapy session 7 where the therapist asked Janice to carefully and intellectually consider the implications for herself of her brother's death.

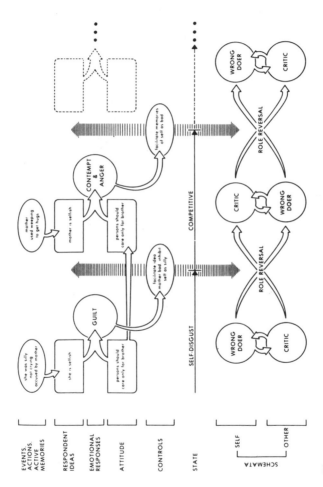

Figure 19A. The Funeral Constellation Described in Step 4 as Leading to Oscillation between Guilt and Anger.

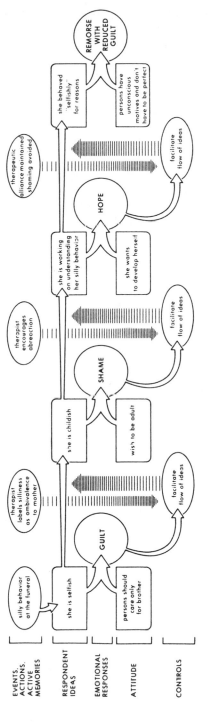

Figure 19B. The Funeral Constellation Leading to Remorse with Reduced Guilt.

The precursors to this moment occurred when the therapist helped her reset the focus, not only on "bad images" of herself, such as laziness, but on bad self-images related in some way to the theme of the death. Immediately after focusing on these issues she reported a dream she had had hours before. She and her brother were saying good-bye because he was going to die. An effort to discuss the dream was made, but the results were superficial and she shifted from a *working* state to the *tra-la-la* state.

The therapist then asked her what the death of her brother meant to her. Her response was intellectual. Recognizing the absence of any authentic self-experience, the therapist pointedly asked her to do what she was already doing, to intellectualize and to rationally explore the meaning to her of her brother's death. That was the reason for his first statement in the excerpt: "But let's be, let's be very rational, very intellectual about it. What does it really mean to you that Sam is dead? [pause] In terms of you?"

The ensuing responses of the patient and the therapist can be placed in tabular form (as in Table 17 of Step 6) to explain shifts in relationships, and are shown here in Table 19.

One inferential meaning of the therapist's remark was that he intended to be more definite in his efforts to find out exactly what she was thinking and feeling. She could have responded cooperatively by deeper contemplation of the meanings, or she could have struggled to go on avoiding the issue. She selected the latter alternative. By saying "My life?" she in effect asked the therapist to explain himself in more detail, or possibly she was attempting to fill in for him what he might have meant. The therapist persisted: "What meanings does it have? Be very reasonable." **Because of his persistence, she altered her role relationship schemata. She could no longer pretend to herself that the immediate situation concerned a person objectively relating an interesting dream in an abstract way to an interested listener. She now experienced herself as a learner who consented to consider the teacher's question, "What does the death really mean to you?" This change caused a shift from the** *tra-la-la* **to the** *hurt but working* **state.**

She began the next moment by saying that it meant nothing: "Well—nothing in, in terms of the things like coming in and giving hugs and stuff." She meant that she would not miss Sam **except** for the hugs. This actually is an undoing couplet: I will not miss anything; I will miss hugs. As she continued, she gradually held more firmly to the concept that the death of her brother did not have major meaning to her: "I don't know [pause] it doesn't mean [pause] it doesn't mean anything that I can put my finger on."

She knew that in response to her statement "It doesn't mean anything," the therapist might either agree or disagree with her. If he disagreed, he would tell her that the brother's death had meanings that she avoided, and she would then experience him as a critic telling her she neglected meanings. He would in effect accuse her of laziness and she would feel defective. She would face entry into either the warded-off state of *self-disgust* or the *competitive* state (where she would reverse roles and criticize the therapist or fend off his criticism). In either event, she would experience the therapist as a critic and, by that, succeed in externalizing her own self-criticism.

As it happened, the therapist did not react in this way. Instead, he endorsed the concept, saying: "Yeah, you know we just looked at it on that level and it doesn't have any big implications for your life on that level at all." By this endorsement the therapist has chosen one of the two possible paths she might have taken if he were silent. That is, **she** might have continued to endorse the death as meaning little to her, or **she** might have undone it by speaking of how the death **did** have meaning for her.

Review of the videotape of this segment showed her in the *hurt but working* state at this point. During some of the long pauses she may even have temporarily entered the *hurt and not working* state. But when the therapist said, "It doesn't have any big implications," she perked up, after looking worried for a moment, and entered the *tra-la-la* state. She said, "In a way it does," in a bright manner. She went on to say, "because it really brings home the reality of things." She went on talking, about having faith in the "reality" (availability) of family members such as her brother. This statement, "In a way it does [have meaning]," disavowed the idea that the death meant little to her. It functioned as a way to avoid continued contemplation of the "it has little meaning" idea.

If she had continued with the "it has little meaning" idea, she would have compared that concept with an enduring attitude that a person ought to care more for others than for herself. She would then experience and criticize herself as selfish, feeling bad that she did not experience enough grief. That type of information processing and that self-image threatens entry into the *self-disgusted* state. She would then experience therapy as a process in which a wrongdoer is exposed to a critic. Her reversal of statements prevented such a feared outcome.

This detailed analysis of interactions shows in microcosm her characteristic use of **externalization** (getting another person to become her critic), **intellectualization** (avoiding emotionally arousing ideas), and **shifting** of meanings (to undo and prevent continuation of a dangerous

Table 19. Microanalysis of Sequential Dialogue: Homesickness Theme

	Literal statements (from therapy hour 7)	Essential statements	Expansion of meanings	Possible reactions	
A.	T: Let's be very rational, very intellectual about it. What does it really mean to you that Sam is dead? In terms of you, what does it (pause)?	T: What intellectual meanings does the event have for you right now?	Let's be more definite about ideas, go ahead with your avoidance of emotion.	P: Contemplate topic. P: Gain time. P: Avoid topic.	●
B.	P: My life?	P: What do you want to know?	1. She is unsure what he means her to do. 2. She doesn't want to follow his line.	T: Repetition, clarification T: Repetition T: Silence T: Interpretation	●
C.	T: What does . . . (pause) what meanings does it have? Be very reasonable.	T: Repeats	As above, let's be definite about what you think.	P: Contemplate meanings. P: Avoid issue.	●
D.	P: Well, nothing in, (pause) in terms of the things like coming in and giving hugs and stuff. . . doesn't mean, (pause) doesn't mean anything that I can put my finger on.	P: It doesn't mean much.	1. It doesn't mean much. 2. She is avoiding meanings	T: Endorse this concept to extend meanings. T: Interpret her disavowal.	●
E.	T: Yeah . . . and it doesn't have any big implications for your life on that level at all.	T: It doesn't mean much to you even on an intellectual level.	1. It doesn't mean much, and you must confront what that implies.	P: Accept and continue on topic, e.g., to express shame that it doesn't mean more to her.	

F. P: In a way it does, it really brings home the reality of things . . . he was **there**. I had the faith . . . now he's not there . . . what's real and what isn't? Is anybody real? Now, all those people that I remember, that I feel close to, that I have this faith in, (pause) maybe they are not real either (pause).	P: It does mean something.	1. She's thought of what it means	T: Confront her with clarifications and extensions of meanings related to independence-homesickness theme. ●
		2. She wants intellectual discussion to avoid emotional reponses.	
		3. She would be bad if the death meant nothing to her.	T: Intepret defense against acknowledging that death elicits little current reaction in her.
		2. You are saying it doesn't mean much to avoid ideas.	P: Disagree.
			P: Agree it doesn't mean much. ●
			P: Find some meanings.
G. T: Yeah well, it symbolizes, then, a larger realm of meanings, which is that the family you were attached to, your childhood and adolescent family, is no longer there for you, 'cause you're no longer a child or an adolescent. You've become independent.	T: You left home, you miss it, but you want to be independent.	You have an active conflict between pining for home and your aim for independence.	P: Accept and continue on topic. ●
			P: Disagree or avoid topic.
H. P: (Long pause) When I get homesick, etc.	P: I miss home.	She is willing to explore homesickness.	T: Explore the independence-homesickness theme. ●

● = Reaction Selected by Respondent.

line of thought). It also shows a nuance of therapy technique. As the segment continued, the therapist chose to go ahead with the shift in meaning she had introduced. As she shifted from saying the event had no impact, she described how she missed her family. There the therapist interpreted her homesickness. This was enough to cause a transition from the *tra-la-la* state, entered by her successful defensive process, back into a *hurt but working* state, where she remained for a time. Later in the hour she verbalized the idea that other members of her family might die and that she would be alone when they (her parents) were dead.

It is possible to diagram the movement of the structure and flow of these ideas, as in Figure 20. The diagram begins with an **act**, the statement by the therapist that he agreed with her that the death had little intellectual meaning for her. Her **respondent idea** was that because it had no meaning she was selfish. That idea, matched against the **enduring attitude** that persons should care more for their brothers than for themselves, leads to emotions labeled in the figure only as guilt, but in fact a medley of feelings that certainly included components of shame. Awareness of the threat of developing feelings of guilt and/or shame evoked anxiety and this anxiety signal motivated her to control the situation. She inhibited the set of ideas having to do with the meaningless aspect of the death, and facilitated ideas about its meaningfulness. Another control, exerted simultaneously, shifted her self-images. As she switched to the alternative that the death had meaning for her, she also shifted to a stronger self-image, strong because she was disagreeing with the therapist, who had just said that the death held little meaning for her. The shift to a stronger position allowed transition from the *hurt but working* state (and the danger of the *self-disgust* state) into the *tra-la-la* state.

She then acted in disagreement with the therapist. This "strength" forced her to go a bit further with ideas about what she **had** lost, so she said the death symbolized the idea that the family she depended on might not really be there for her. When she matched this **respondent** idea with the **attitude** that she needed ties to her parents, she tended toward sad feelings. To encourage development of this train of thought, the therapist then labeled the warded-off feelings and ideas by interpretation of the homesickness. This encouraged her to facilitate these ideas. She could again safely enter the *working* state, in which the guiding self-image is that of learner. With threat, she would return to the *tra-la-la* state. She could also shift between ideas of whether or not the death has meanings and so accomplish undoing of threats. Controlled settings for associations at a general level accomplished both intellectualization and isolation. Additionally, she could reduce threatening emotions by

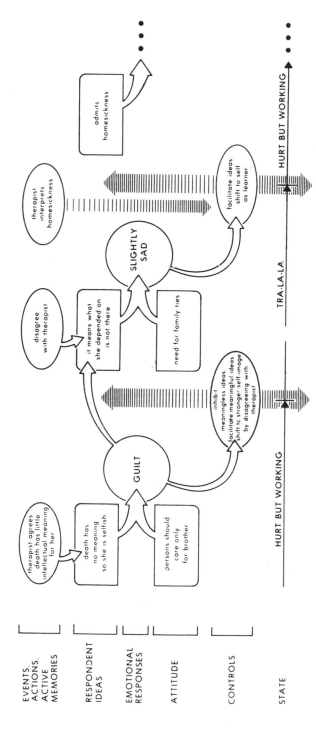

Figure 20. State Transitions and the Homesickness Constellation.

EVENTS,
ACTIONS,
ACTIVE
MEMORIES

RESPONDENT
IDEAS

EMOTIONAL
RESPONSES

ATTITUDE

CONTROLS

STATE

therapist agrees
death has little
intellectual meaning
for her

death has
no meaning
so she is selfish

persons should
care only
for brother

GUILT

inhibit
meaningless ideas,
facilitate meaningful ideas,
shift to stronger self-image
by disagreeing with
therapist

disagree
with therapist

it means what
she depended on
is not there

need for family ties

SLIGHTLY
SAD

therapist
interprets
homesickness

admits
homesickness

facilitate ideas,
shift to self
as learner

HURT BUT WORKING   TRA-LA-LA   HURT BUT WORKING

undoing guilt with sadness and she could reduce sad feelings by feeling slightly guilty or ashamed. This oscillation at a process level can also be seen at a structural level as shifting between the strong and weak self-images. **Controls effect the oscillations by modifying both ideas and self-images or role relationships.**

Through application, then, to just a few phrases, the previously described patterns of transition between states, role relationships, and characteristic controls seem to be pertinent and to have explanatory power. Microanalysis is a useful check on configurational analysis.

SUMMARY

Analysis of change as it occurs through transformation of information involves the most inferential aspects of configurational analysis. It is the step most assisted by the work of prior steps. A problematic constellation of ideas, feelings, and controls will already have been described in Step 4, and related to the various states, self-images, and relationship models of the person as elucidated in surrounding steps. The change period is then examined in terms of phases. The status of the constellation in each phase is examined first. Then the reasons for observed differences in status are examined as they relate to the input of information that alters controls. Such input is as varied as human behavior but the interventions and techniques of the therapist in relation to the defenses and initiatives of the patient are central.

The status of sets of ideas and emotion as they affect thinking consciously or unconsciously is an important facet of examining the status of the selected constellation in the various phases of the change period. Equally important is the status of sequential organization for working through ideas. That is, there is a natural property of the mind, its intrinsic tendency to work over and work out incongruities, conflicts, and problems; it is a self-organizing, self-regulating, and self-healing system that is not only influenced by interventions. Internal controls and control limitations may frustrate the optimal play of these intrinsic properties. Interventions from the therapist, whether interpretations or medications to correct electrochemical imbalances, can be examined for their effects on the internal controls of the patient. Relevant patterns are first described macroscopically, and then explanations can be tested for explanatory power by the type of microanalytic procedure described in this chapter.

The relative solution of one problem contributes to other problems. Various constellations of ideas, feelings, and controls will interact in the generally accepted overdetermined process of human psychology. That is why the actual steps of a given configurational analysis will always be individualized to person, time, and context. But these general principles of observation should apply across most situations. New theories of change process will then provide additional facets for such observation. **We are aware of possibilities, but as of now, we know surprisingly little about what can change, how fast change can occur, and what intervention can accomplish what changes in what kind of person.** And, when change does occur during therapy, we do not know if it lasts, or if it is only an alteration during the therapy period. This final problem is the focus of the remaining three steps of configurational analysis.

III

Description of Outcome

The final review of states, self-concepts, role relationship models, and information processing is from the viewpoint of outcome. The ideal information would be derived from follow-up interviews. These ensuing steps can, however, be carried forward even when data from follow-up are unavailable, with data from later points of the therapy used instead.

While not essential, follow-up data are extremely useful for the observation of positive changes that do not emerge until the person has had time to live through solutions to previous problems. Follow-up is also useful in examining the progress of those positive changes that are due to the existence of the therapeutic situation itself, and that may have dissipated after that situation terminated. Finally, the end of therapy carries its own sources of turbulence. Separation from the therapist and reactions to the realization that "this is it for now" may cause temporary state alterations that would confuse both patient and therapist in estimating the stability of state changes that had been effected before the termination phase.

CHAPTER EIGHT

Alteration in the Frequency and Quality of States

Step 8. States: *Describe outcome in terms of changes in signs, symptoms, and states. Include discussion of interaction of situational factors with change, including family, social, environmental, and neurobiological systems. Discuss new states, state cycles, and state triggers. Use labels from Steps 2 and 5.*

The ideal outcome is marked by a cessation of problem states and the substitution of adaptive, self-actualized, satisfying states. Such ideal goals are seldom the outcome of change processes. More frequently, in a good outcome, problem states are attenuated; they change form and frequency and blend with other states, but do not totally disappear. If a person begins therapy with anxiety attacks and a good outcome occurs, he no longer has anxiety attacks after therapy, but continues to experience moments of uneasiness, tension, or dread under certain circumstances. When he does feel anxious, the state is less intense and experienced in the same way as other states. A person may markedly improve from a condition of continuous depression and still have moments of gloom, morbid self-reflection, and sadness without feeling severe emotional pain or loss of control. Since outcomes are not an all-or-nothing phenomenon, an analysis of states must include attention to qualitative as well as quantitative alterations.

The entry into and exit from states is often a vital aspect of a person's subjective sense of being in or out of control. We can then proceed to a discussion of the increase or decrease in tolerance for stressful events in terms of state stability and likelihood of state transitions, and the description and evaluation of entry and exit qualities. For example, a person may note that he no longer plunges into sharply different states but flows between moods almost imperceptibly.

Summation should include the making of value judgments and an appraisal of the total picture of state frequencies, qualities, and cycles in terms of worthwhile and harmful aspects. For example, at outcome a person may no longer have a state characterized by out-of-control hostile acts, and the experience of frighteningly monstrous thoughts and emotional pain. But he may be on maintenance drugs that leave him feeling apathetic and drained, with mild muscle spasms of the mouth and tongue. The expense of any cure must be stated as objectively as possible.

Illustration

In the pretherapy period, Janice felt her greatest emotional pain during periods of *self-disgust* and her most chronic dull pain in the depressed, *hurt but not working* state. As noted in the statement of problems, her self-report of depression declined nicely. The states of *self-disgust* occurred less frequently toward the end of therapy. During the year that followed therapy, they were also less frequent, as indicated by the evaluation interview at the end of that year. During the posttherapy period there were other signs of positive change in other states. She *cried* less often, and was in the *hurt-and-not-working* state less often. She spent more time in a *working* state, during which she felt less hurt. In addition her *competitive* state was somewhat more in control and the quality of this state changed. When in this state she did not yield to impulsive outbursts of temper but was able to continue effective interchanges with the challenging person. The result was improved work performance and more rewards from her colleagues.

There were no new states noted. Her *tra-la-la* state remained frequent, although the quality of this state changed. She experienced herself as somewhat more authentic, a movement in the direction of an ideal *competent* state she was not yet able to stabilize.

In general, then, differentiation between states was not as clear because the extreme qualities of states were lessened. This may be a general positive effect of relatively successful therapies. Janice felt transitions between states to be less passive and happenstance. She was aware of her states and to some extent could control herself at points of likely transition. For example, during the first evaluation interview, three months after termination of therapy, she said: "I feel like from the therapy and from the time that has gone by, uh, I've reached a lot more of an equilibrium and even now, when I'm in a mood, I can see a reason for it." Later in that interview, after the evaluator asked her to comment specifically on her moods, she said, "I feel like it's more of an equilibrium. It's kind of settled into a comfortable, fairly content thing. And it goes up and down from there, always returning to . . . to there, instead of going like this [waves her arms about] without a return to anything!"

Her fear that the improvement might be transient is reflected in the following comment on her relationship with a supervisor at work: "I feel like last spring I had so much trouble with the woman that I was working under partially because of that emotional instability. I mean, I just couldn't react safely to people. And this year I'm just crossing my fingers out of, like, a superstitious fear that it might happen again. I'm working under a different woman as a group worker and it's going fantastic. I feel that part of it is that I'm more confident and I'm doing a better job. I mean, this woman last year, her complaints were not entirely groundless, even though I reacted at first as if they were. But, um, I feel like this year, I'm just more together and able to give more, and be more aware and on top of things. I don't know how long it will last. Just being in the same room with her still kind of shakes me up. I mean, I look for undertones and words between the lines just when we say hello to each other."

She also said, "I was out of control [before therapy] and there were all these signs and I'm . . . I'm seeing that in her now [a friend who is out of control] and it reminds me, at the same time, it makes me feel really good for not being there [out of control] anymore."

She kept her perspective on states over the year that followed therapy, and her confidence in her control increased. For example, in the evaluation interview close to the one-year point after treatment she said, "I've just become a lot stronger . . . [even] when I feel tired and depressed . . . I can see that as temporary."

To summarize, then, there was no dramatic change in terms of new states. A positive outcome was evident in the reduced frequency of entry into the states of *self-disgust*, *crying*, and *hurt and not working*. The quality of the *hurt but working* state changed so that the hurt quality diminished. The quality of the *competitive* state changed, with a less strident struggle to avoid submission by becoming dominant. The quality of the *tra-la-la* state changed, with less feeling of pretending and lack of authenticity. Overall, the states were less discrete, the extremes were reduced, and there was more control of transitions. She had not yet achieved the desired state where she would have a sense of **personal**

integrity, competence, and **mutuality**, but felt closer to that goal. She had not removed herself from the danger of *self-disgust*, but felt more confident and distant from that threat.

In overall judgment of outcome as measured by states, she seemed no worse, and generally better off. Her state of not working on developmental plans had diminished in both frequency and intensity, and also her state of self-disgust was more securely avoided. The outcome was not that of ideal goals, however, since she had not yet reached a developmental point where she could feel securely competent.

CHAPTER NINE

Modification of Self-Concepts and Role Relationship Models

Step 9. Interpersonal Behavioral Patterns, Self Concepts, and Role Relationship Models: *Describe the outcome in terms of changes and persistence of maladaptive interpersonal behavioral patterns and patterns of self-regard. Include an analysis of changes in personal contacts, family, social structure, and situational opportunities that may have played a role in the changes noted. Infer the changes and developments in person schemata that may have led to these alterations in behavior. Include modifications in enduring attitudes, value hierarchies, and personal agendas.*

The ultimate test of any durable change in relationship models is to be found in the patterns of behavior and conscious experience that continue after the therapy period. The person should be able to do things differently or to experience them internally as qualitatively different. The main patterns will have already been identified for the baseline and change periods. Now the task will be to state analogous patterns for the outcome period.

BACKGROUND

The conflictual or impaired self-concepts and relationship themes can be discussed as they apply to a variety of positive and negative outcomes. For example, suppose a person complained initially of being depressed about his inability to continue a heterosexual relationship beyond the first few dates because he becomes excessively deadened and withdrawn. A most valuable outcome would manifest itself by continued, animated, interesting, sexually potent, loving, intimate attachment. A negative outcome would involve continued depression with avoidance of all options for beginning new relationships. A lateral solution such as attachment to a much older person in a dependent relationship might relieve the depression but be judged as a "valuable false solution" rather than a positive outcome to a specifically defined problem (Malan, 1976a). Such value judgments can even be reliably quantified (Kaltreider, DeWitt, Weiss, and Horowitz, 1981; Weiss, DeWitt, Kaltreider, and Horowitz, 1985; Horowitz, Marmar, Weiss *et al.*, 1986).

Evaluation of outcome in terms of self-concepts and role relationship models must take into consideration the continuous motion of life. Every period of life brings new demands; maturational unfolding does not end with adolescence, and culture shifts undermine or reinforce certain roles. It is never possible to say for sure that a given alteration in behavior was due to a particular change force; **every outcome will be pluridetermined**. One must also be wary of ideals that may be illusory markers against which to compare actual outcomes. Absolute tranquillity, the absence of unconscious processes, the nullification of transference potential, and complete self-actualization have been touted as outcomes of therapy. One should not diminish the value of some really satisfying modification in behavior because it is not equal in kind to unsubstantiated claims or longed-for, unreachable goals such as these.

METHOD

The outcome period is examined for interpersonal behavior patterns and conscious self-experiences that can be compared in some way to the patterns and experiences described in earlier relationship steps. What has been developed futher? What has regressed? What has ceased? What is new? What has stayed the same? For all these questions, the usual answers when change is positive is that some forms, already present like seeds, will have flourished and differentiated, not changed completely to something else or grown up without precursors. Dreaded self-concepts and role relationship models remain present in some form of memory, but they become less common, less feared, less easily triggered, less global or diffuse, and descriptions should aim at such qualifications.

The traditional method for establishing contrasts is to state the situation before and after a treatment, and to contemplate the difference.

The methods described in Chapter 3 for defining self-concepts and role relationship models are suitable for this purpose. This traditional method is helped by use of an additional contrast. **One can compare the situation before and the situation after the treatment in terms of the distance between the self-concepts of the patient and his ideal goals.** Was he closer to or further from his goals after therapy? Did his goals change? One can repeat this for ingrained threats: Was the person closer to or more remote from his dreaded self-concepts at the conclusion of therapy? Did his fears change?

The statements can also be made in terms of integration of traits into the self-concept. For example, suppose a person had as a goal the ability to become independent of the criticism of others and to be able to criticize himself. Before therapy, a given criticism may have been experienced by him as if coming from a harsh parental judge. After therapy, the criticism may have been experienced by him as a softer inner voice, more like a self-remonstration against an impulsive deviation from personal standards.

Illustration

Janice had brief treatment only 12 hours in duration. The limitation of the data, as compared with data from a long-term psychoanalytic psychotherapy, precludes a comprehensive view of self and other schemata. Nevertheless, it was possible in Chapter 3 to describe a repertoire of recurrent self-images and complementary images of others. The play of these self-concepts and roles during therapy was reviewed in Chapter 6. As noted, an important adaptive self-concept was herself as learner. It was used in the role relationship model of the therapeutic alliance, with the therapist as teacher and model of something of potential value for her. Unlike her image of her mother, she saw the therapist as not discouraging her own individuation by fostering dependent attachment. The principal change in self-images, in terms of outcome, was stabilization of this self-concept and of the learner–teacher role relationship for use outside of therapy. In other words, the gains made in formation of the therapeutic alliance continued into the posttherapy period. She was able to continue to develop her own self-concept without being too much like or too rebelliously different from her mother. While she had progressed, she had not accomplished this life task at final evaluation 1 year after therapy.

On what grounds are such assertions advanced? She manifested changes in interpersonal behavior and self-experiences. She remained away from home and continued her attempts to improve her career. She made efforts to establish ties to new women friends. She was able to move away from Phillip without feeling intolerably lonely. By the time of the 1-year follow-up she was well into recognition of the loss of her relationship with her brother through the normal healing process of mourning. Some of these assertions of outcome can now be examined in greater detail.

Stabilization of her self-concept as a person learning to become more competent, creative, and womanly meant she became less vulnerable to images of herself as defective, bad, or as a harsh and superior critic of others. It meant less pretense at having already reached her ideal and less vulnerability to shame if and when this pretense failed. Her stabilized self-concept and models of relationships manifested themselves in reduced maladaptive behavior. During the year after therapy, she was able to tolerate subordinate positions at work without feeling as degraded or behaving as maladaptively. She was able to get closer to another woman without feeling submerged or smothered. She was able to break up with Phillip without feeling excessively needy, lonely, and deprived. She was able to tolerate the absence of the therapeutic alliance without relapse into depression.

These gains put her at a greater distance from her fears of stagnation, defectiveness, and dependency, but when seen 1 year after therapy, it was clear that these gains fell short of her ideals. The outcome 1 year after therapy was good, but not as good as it could have been. She did not maintain the weight loss begun during therapy, she had not arrived at her full potential for mutuality, and she had not developed her creativity and work capacities to the degree she desired. At the end of therapy she felt that she was again on her way but was uncertain of the stability of these gains. As a result of her own efforts over the year, she had an increased sense of confidence and stability in herself as a person learning and gaining from life experiences.

These statements are illustrated with excerpts from the last therapy hour and from the two evaluation sessions 3 and 11 months after therapy. In the last treatment hour she reviewed her gains and spoke of her fear that the loss of the therapeutic alliance would mean a regression to apathy and depression:

P: Oh, yeah. When you reminded me two or three sessions ago that we only had a few weeks left, I was really horrified. [Pause] Um, "Oh, God, no. We can't stop, I'll be lost and . . ." Like I said, the long-distance phone call feeling. We have . . . we have to accomplish something in each session, and then we can point to it and say, "This is what we accomplished" [pause]. I think it's also when I started thinking, uh, maybe I'd like to try it by myself for a while.

In the first evaluation session three months after therapy, Janice reported that she was still living with Phillip and that this depressed her. She had not maintained the weight loss that began during therapy, but in other respects she felt generally more in control of herself. She experienced less of a sense of herself as defective and seldom had recourse to the compensatory grandiosity of superwoman fantasies. She was pleased by this change, but concerned about maintaining it.

Evaluator (E): Do you feel like your life changed much during or after the period that you were in therapy?
P: Yes, I do, a lot. I feel, um [long pause] like when I came in and for most of the time that I was in therapy, I was really upset about a lot of things and shaky an—and unstable. And I, I felt very, very out of control. Like, moods would come and I had no idea where they had come from or what to do about them. Kind of falling over cliffs all the time. And I don't feel that way anymore. I feel like from the therapy and from the time that has gone by, uh, I've reached a lot more of an equilibrium and even now, when I'm in a mood, I can see a reason for it and I mean I don't feel like superwoman or anything but. . . .
E: But you're feeling more in control of your feelings.
P: I am. An— . . . and in my . . . of my environment. And I feel like last spring, I had so much trouble with the woman that I was working under, partially because of that emotional instability. I mean, I just couldn't react safely to people, and this year I'm just crossing my fingers out of, like, superstitious fear that it might happen again. I'm working under a different woman and it's going fantastic.

The process of improvement in her self-concepts and self-experiences continued and at the second evaluation session 11 months after therapy, she said, "I feel a lot more in control of myself and of my life than I did then." She had been "not just thrown by his [her brother's] death, but just powerless in general. Like, everything kind of fell apart and I feel like I'm. . . . I know what direction I'm going in [now]. I have plans, and I'm more able to deal with daily crises and stuff and, in fact, I'm dealing with a major crisis in a way that I'm feeling pretty good about. The major crisis was that I'm leaving my, the guy that I've been living with."

She had gained sufficient self-confidence to separate, and she went on affirming this:

E: But even in crises you still have some sense of control.
P: I, right. I feel like I, you know, I, er, even though, even when I'm aware of being **really** confused or **really** depressed, um, I have, a, this a— you know, a little more sense of me-ness and of liking the me and, um, just since talking to you and making this last appointment I have obviously been kind of thinking what's happening, and I've just been really pleased about it.

Later, while talking specifically about the decision to leave Phillip, the evaluating clinician confronted her with her previous worry about that relationship:

E: What's your sense of what's changed? I remember the last time I talked to you, it was your feeling that you were a little uncomfortable about that relationship with Phillip, that you didn't want to examine it 'cause you were afraid of what you might find.
P: Hmmmm. I don't know. Possibly, I'm feeling so much better about myself that I don't need as much security, and I'm more able to face the things I don't like about the relationship.

She also described the distance from her ideal. For example, she said that she is not yet capable of an extended relationship:

P: I demand a lot out of any relationship. I mean this is one thing that bugs me, is I feel like I'm a failure at relationships. I can never have one that lasts for longer than a year. I'll probably be an old maid all my life 'cause I can't live with people, just impossible. And I, I say that kind of facetiously.
E: But those are thoughts you've been having.
P: But those are thoughts I've been having, yeah. And, um, anyway, one of the things I do want to change is I want to be able to learn, not so much to be more objective, but to, uh, to know what to do with all my emotions and my pressure and to, to be able to take things easy a little bit more. Like, if I, if I hadn't been demanding so much of him, I wouldn't have been so bothered. Of course, you can say that a different way, you could say if I hadn't cared so much for him, I wouldn't have been so bothered. I mean if I didn't give a damn about him, I wouldn't give a damn what he did.

Such concerns led her to decide to seek more therapy. She spoke of mixed feelings about this; she wished to avoid any dependency or subordination. She said:

> I've been thinking. Maybe a group would be better than a one-person thing, because it would be less like, I don't know, I guess, like, therapy or going to a shrink. And there'd be the perceptions of other people. It wouldn't be the choice between **your** opinion and **my** opinion or something like that. Yeah. I really liked Dr. Jones's objectivity. I, I felt myself being able to just be myself instead of, like, trying to impress him or trying to win his sympathy or anything. And I imagine a group wouldn't be able to do that as much. On the other hand, one of the things I want right now is to find out what I believe about a lot of things, you know, whether I actually believe this or whether I've just been kind of conditioned to believe it, by (a) my parents or (b) my peers. And, you know, what I really want. And if I have a bunch of different opinions, then maybe I can use bunches of people as sounding boards and, either in agreement or in contradiction, and find out what I think.

One may infer from these statements that there has been some small gain in her self-concept as completely independent, but that there is residual worry, or a sense of conflict in role relationships around the theme of becoming independent. In other words, a central problem theme before therapy had a similar but somewhat more advanced configuration after therapy. No major personality reorganization or structural change had occurred in this brief therapy. She was not blocked, however, and one could be optimistic about further advances.

SUMMARY

The series of self-concepts described for the pretherapy period can be compared with the series of self-concepts as experienced or manifested during the posttherapy period. The qualities of self-concept, the sense of selfhood, the coherence over time, and the degree of felt control and valuation will all be important to note, as will any increase in separation from others. Role relationships can be discussed not only in terms of mental models, experienced and reported or inferred, but by observing changes in capability and transactions. Even if real transactions have not changed, outcome valuation may be positive if inner aspects have altered. For example, a person who has depressive states because of perfectionist standards of self may feel better with softening of ideal self-concepts and less incongruity between real and ideal self-experiences. In other words, individualized outcome assessment in terms of self and relationship issues must strike a balance in relying on external affairs and internal experiences.

CHAPTER TEN

Change in Ideational Constellations and Information-Processing Style

Step 10. Information Processing

A. Themes: *Describe outcome in terms of changes or shifts in the themes described in Step 4. Relate these modifications to changes in emotional responses, memories, and fantasies. Include comments about increased or decreased scope of life purposes or plans.*

B. Habitual Styles: *Describe changes in coping, defensive, or conceptual styles noted in Steps 4 and 7.*

Change in the status of ideas can be described using the original topographic model of Freud (1900/1953a). **The status of ideas can be specified in terms of accessibility to consciousness and actions of volitional effort. As an outcome of therapy, memories or ideas once warded off by unconscious controls despite conscious efforts to retrieve them now may be available for contemplation.** This change in ideational status is not simply an increase in "insight," unless that term is given broader meaning. Such change not only involves retrieval of repressed ideas, but formulation of new meanings and associational connections that can be explained in terms of specific forms and contents.

Shifts in the basic premises used to appraise the past, present and future are also important and closely related to self-concepts and role relationship models. Here these may be discussed as injunctions or rules such as "you have to be perfect to be loved," "if one person gets loved more, another gets loved less," or "bad thoughts cause death." Altered power of such injunctions, less repetition, or prevalence, are changes that may be noted (Beck, 1976).

Emotions elicited with expression of ideas are among relevant qualities to be described. Themes that were once accompanied by turbulent emotional feelings may now be thought about in a quieter mood. Ideas once expressed with intellectual detachment may now be formed with enriched feeling or passionate commitment. The quality and intensity of emotions may change.

The relation of ideas and feelings to intention is also an important quality to describe when reporting change. Ideas that were intrusive and disrupted concentration may now be less peremptory. What was then unthinkable may now be contemplated. The person may be able to both recall a traumatic memory and put it out of mind. He may be able to relate to his mother without having unbidden bad images of her, or to recognize a disliked trait without overgeneralizing its meaning.

Change may also be described in qualitative differences in thought itself. New abilities to organize sequences of rational and coherent meaning may have been developed. A person may have learned to think in visual images, or to do so in some different way. He may have learned to sense and use bodily experiences once ignored. Bodily communications once transmitted unknowingly or avoided may now be part of known and deliberate expression.

Changes in the quality of experiences might include an increased sense of vitality, a new grounding of awareness in reality, changes in associational abilities, increased or decreased creativity, increased or decreased capacity to enter altered states of consciousness, and changed ability to plan and carry out actions. The ability to think through plans in moments of frustration is one of the more frequent positive outcomes noted from work in psychotherapy.

Among the most important considerations will be inference about modifications of habitual styles for control of thought and emotion. Since defense must be considered in interaction with sources of both internal and external stress, such inferences will be difficult to make. If stress is low, then the person may be less defensive. Controls will be less apparent to the clinical observer without any necessary change in the person's cognitive style or capacity. On the other hand, changes in cognitive style that lessen defenses of avoidance and distortion may help a person to cope with and so reduce stress, but may also encourage him to take on more challenging life tasks. The greater challenge may leave him at a level of stress similar to the pretherapy period. Assessment of change in defensive style means a complex consideration of the goals set by the person and the degree of stress present.

To recapitulate, Step 10 describes patterns at outcome in terms of altered status of information in conscious experience, altered basic premises and attitudes, altered styles of awareness and attention deployment, and general changes in regulatory patterns. The difficult inferences required are rendered easier by the identification of important themes in the earlier steps, and by information from the pretherapy period and during the processes of change.

Illustration

For Janice, the main warded-off constellations of ideas were centered on themes of her present status and future aims as an independent person, particularly in relation to her brother's death, her return home, and interactions with her parents at the funeral. At treatment onset she was unable to mourn for her brother. She felt she was floundering and at sea, with impaired ability to think through her plans, and with conflicted feelings about returning home or staying away, about separation, and about identification with her mother.

One outcome of therapy was the availability of these themes to her conscious thinking, although they were not yet completely worked through to the point of making definite choices or plans of action. Integration and resolution of these conflicts would be possible only when a more mature and secure self-image had been established, a process under way but not completed. Many relevant memories and associations could now be consciously contemplated with appropriate emotional expression. While it is implied that this constellation was not completely worked through, her movement toward this goal was significant and important. Indeed, despite the difficulties in focusing on it early in therapy, she felt that her reactions to her brother's death were the feelings most resolved at the end of treatment. She said in the last therapy hour:

> It's kind of funny. One of the things I feel most finished about is what I said I came in here for, which is about Sam's death. I mean all this time I've come to be much more accepting about my feelings about his death. I still dream about him, but I've been glad dreaming about him. I've been glad to be getting flashes of him, because it hasn't been with that feeling of avoidance, instant rejection, and everything.

Toward the end of treatment and in the later evaluation sessions, she seemed, in a general way, more aware of her communications, more open to ideas, and richer in terms of experienced and expressed emotionality. These changes could be due simply to reduced frequency in state changes and to a lessening in intensity of her depressive moods and *hurt* states. It was not assessed as due to any major revisions of cognitive capacity.

Her defensive style also seemed to shift, but this could be accounted for by the changes in state and reduction in stress noted above. There was insufficient evidence for assertion of any change in her style of processing information. She began with a diverse defensive style. She used inhibition to accomplish unconscious repression and conscious suppression. To avoid experiencing painful affect, she used disavowal, intellectualization, depersonification, generalization, externalization, and switching maneuvers. She used these defenses less in the last therapy sessions, but this change was due to an increased stress tolerance provided by the therapeutic alliance, and to the now expected interventions of the therapist to counteract her avoidances. This reduction in controls allowed her to integrate the memory of the funeral, to begin to react to her brother's death, and to contemplate her conflicts around strivings for independence. It cannot, however, be taken as evidence of enduring change in the general quality of her defensive and coping styles.

The only possible changes in cognitive style, with scant evidence for such inference, were observed in the adoption of an objective stance, modeled in part after that of the therapist, which allowed a more conscious use of the regulatory operations that were previously imposed unconsciously upon her thought process. In other words, the final evaluation was that she still used the defenses she began with, whenever the need for defense was present, but did so with slightly more conscious control.

Illustrations of these assertions about changes in ideas and control habits can be found in her statements during the follow-up evaluation sessions. In the first evaluation session three months after therapy, she indicated an increase in the insight she had gained into her responses at the funeral. For example, she said, "I just . . . wouldn't cry. It was because I didn't want to play their game. I didn't want to be sucked back in. I'm still—I'm still trying to—to be apart and be myself. And so I can't [pause] I couldn't really let go."

This increased ability to talk about previously warded-off ideas is shown in relation to customary defensive operations in the following excerpt from the evaluation 1 year after therapy.

E: It's striking that you're talking so much about your current life and your future plans and that you really haven't mentioned your brother's death.
P: My brother. Um, I'm going home in August, and, we're going to go to his grave and plant flowers and I find that thought uncomfortable. I don't know [an inhibitory operation] if, if you know, because it'll be final, uh, because I'm afraid I'll be embarrassed in front of my family [statement of the threat], you know I mean, it's gonna be a sentimental, emotional occasion.
E: How would you be embarrassed?

P: Oh. God. What if I cry too much? What if I don't cry? [Switching operation]
     You know, I . . . it's this . . . it's this thing, uh, I don't know [inhibitions].
     I guess I want to feel the right thing on that occasion and I'm afraid I won't.

The last statement, "I want to feel the right thing on that occasion, and
I'm afraid I won't," presented ideas but also incorporated a switching
maneuver. At an underlying level she was afraid she would feel too
much, or experience the wrong emotions. She reduced this threat with
the idea of having very little feeling, and went on to the complementary
fear that she would be numb, would again feel too little and repeat her
withdrawal at the funeral. This type of switching was again illustrated
when she talked of future therapy. She said she wanted group therapy:
"The picture I have in my mind is kind of a feminist-oriented group of
women, because one of the things I am really concerned about is how
I relate to men. Maybe having some men around would be helpful in
that, in that area." That is, she switched between saying she wanted to
be in a group with other women and in a mixed group. A desire to avoid
an individual therapist indicated, perhaps, the residual presence of fears
of surrendering her independence to the ideas or controls of another
person.

SUMMARY

Working through of the conflicted ideas of the homesickness, independence, and funeral constellations was useful and partial. As an outcome of this brief therapy, there was little change in general character
as seen in cognitive style and in defensive and coping strategies. There
was an apparent shift away from the use of disavowal, externalization,
and extremes of intellectualization about the problem constellations. She
was able to gradually dose herself with threatening ideas by continued
use of inhibitory and switching processes. There were possible gains in
the use of such conscious coping strategies as doing, deciding, being
objective, analyzing situations, and making step-by-step decisions. These
changes were due to reduced stress from working through memories of
Sam's death, his funeral, and the identity crisis heightened by these
events.

For the therapy illustrated above, the testing of the therapist and
the eventual development of a therapeutic alliance seemed to be the
predominant process that caused improvement. To her, it meant that
in psychotherapy she could work on organizing her immediate life, on
relating to a person who was seen as helpful but not too intrusive or

demanding of identification or subordination. She could bear being helped by a person not overly concerned or overly attached. The relationship encouraged her, allowed her to begin to resolve her responses to the death of her brother, and sustained her temporarily in an identity crisis, allowing continued personal efforts toward independence, attachments to new figures, and learning of skills.

The most important gain in her self-concept came from realizing that she could not only undertake and participate in the therapy, but could also tolerate the separation from it and from the therapist. These ideational processes led to a major shift within the variety of her available self- and object images, a shift back in the direction of experiencing herself as independent and competent. Continued work on her own, or in future therapy, would be necessary to solidify this goal of personal development.

This concludes the presentation of the ten steps of configurational analysis. The next section describes its application using other cases as illustrations.

IV

Applications of Configurational Analysis

The ten steps of configurational analysis have been outlined and illustrated. This approach to examining and describing change can be used as a tool in teaching, in research, and in direct service to patients undergoing psychotherapy. Shorter versions and partial steps are feasible and useful. The next three chapters discuss such application of the method.

CHAPTER ELEVEN

Use of Configurational Analysis in Teaching

In a training situation, one can more quickly cover a broad overview and then deal specifically and at length with one issue and one or more steps of configurational analysis. The overview indicates the particular facet of explanation to be explored and presents an idea of how it articulates with other levels of explanation, even when these levels are not explicated.

Configurational analysis can be used with boldness, simplicity, and a willingness to blunder through, without the detail, complexity, and microanalytic approach that characterized the earlier presentation of the method. It is particularly rewarding to describe cases after completion of treatment. For other cases, a segment or a step or two of the configurational analysis format can be applied in more depth and detail. This chapter will provide three new case studies as illustrations. One is a case review, and two are detailed but partial studies.

First, a relatively unpolished review of a case will be presented. It follows each of the ten steps without becoming extensive and illustrates how formulations can be made during a review of process notes.

Process notes are invaluable as a source of information when such reviews of a therapeutic process are conducted. We have found, in supervising trainees, that such notes often dwell too extensively on the sequential flow of contents and tend to ignore process observations. To counteract this tendency, the following set of additional subheadings provides a useful format for writing process notes after each interview, when one intends to use configurational analysis to conceptualize or clarify change processes.

1. States and events occurring before this hour (e.g., since last interview).

2. States and events during this interview.
3. Contents, inferences, and interactions about self-images and role relationships (include past, current, and patient-therapist relationships).
4. Expressions and interactions around other ideas, feelings, styles, defenses, symptoms, problem solving, practice, and new awareness.
5. Interventions (including possible errors, prescriptions, "techniques").
6. Working formulations (interpretations not made, diagnostic and prognostic speculations, predictions).

CONNIE: A SAMPLE CASE REVIEW FOLLOWING COMPLETION OF PSYCHOTHERAPY

Identifying Information and Event Structure

Connie is a 28-year-old single white female, supporting herself on unemployment assistance while retraining for a new, more fulfilling career. Until a week before entering therapy she had been living with a man, but when first seen, she was living with other friends. She was self-referred because of distress about intrusive crying and depressed feelings related to the death of her father 5 weeks earlier. After evaluation she was seen in brief, time-limited psychotherapy. She gave informed consent for recordings and use of information for scientific and teaching purposes.

1. Problem List. She complained of intrusive episodes of crying, which she felt bad about and attempted to stifle or conceal. During conversations with others she was unable to follow the thread of meaning and instead became dazed. After the death of her father her creative work stopped. She was frightened by these symptoms because they seemed to lead into states where she had less and less control over herself. She was preoccupied with thoughts of death and, in addition to the sudden outbursts of sadness, had difficulty concentrating and an overall sense of lack of purpose and direction in her life. Most of these symptoms had disappeared at the time of the first follow-up interview, 3 months after the end of therapy.

Formulated complaints included fear of an intense mourning reaction that would leave her too depleted to carry on. This operated in the context of an unresolved Oedipus complex characterized by a repetitive reenactment of the search to establish an idealized relationship with an older man. In actual behavior this led to a pattern of frequent disruptive love affairs for which she would select cold and remote men, in a vain attempt to teach them to love her. Another problem was her inability to arrive at an adult understanding of her relationship with her father, an issue exacerbated by his death and meanings associated with it. She was especially unable to understand the meaning of various episodes in which her father had rejected her. She was unable to experience any resentment toward him for rejecting her, without having to distort the meaning of the good relationships that she remembered. This led to feelings of confusion about who she was and who he was and how she should appropriately respond to his death. This problem was intensified by Connie's inability to know where she stood in terms of identification with her mother, except for a relatively imperative need to be unlike her. She, her father, and her siblings shared a view of the mother as a person who gave way easily to messy, out-of-control, emotional episodes of rage and depression.

At the first follow-up interview, Connie was seen as having progressed to a level of normal grief, with ability to know and tolerate feelings of resentment toward her father as well as to simultaneously know the extent of her love and feelings of loss for that relationship. No signs of decisive change were noted in resolution of the other formulated problems, other than partial insight into their existence. It was anticipated that more information about these problems would be available 1 year after therapy than was observable at the 3-month follow-up.

2. *State Analysis.* The most upsetting problem state was characterized by uncontrolled and *intrusive crying*. There were other states used as defenses against this one, such as increased *sleeping*. The *dazed and distracted* state was seen as a problem but was apparently defensive, and preferable to the uncontrolled and painful crying experiences. There were also *high-pressured* states in which she felt "as if crazy."

3. *Relationships.* She was vulnerable to defective self-concepts, especially around her vocational identity or sense of competence. She had followed her father's line of development in completing college, and in obtaining work as a very minor bank executive. She felt that this was a dead end, and her lack of more advanced skills made her feel relatively worthless. She left her job so that she could have a period in which to reorient her values and develop her skills. She was in the midst of this period when her father died. His death meant the interruption of her plan in which he would come to see that she was a worthwhile person, revise the rejection she had felt for the past 5 years, and so restore an early adolescent relationship of mutual admiration.

This rejection of her was mysterious and unexplained even before his death. In fact, the last time Connie had seen him was part of an effort by her to regain the positive attachment of her earlier adolescence or at least to find out the reasons for his neglect and remoteness. She saw her father as a cold, selfish man who had, in a way, tricked and used her in his eventual divorce from her mother and then neglected and no longer needed her when he married a woman much younger than himself with whom he then had a child. She experienced scorn and then felt herself to be either defective or unfairly rejected.

She was unable to identify with her mother, although she had lost some of the basis for her identification with her father and his projections of what she ought to be. Her father wanted the divorce supposedly because of the mother's episodic, out-of-control rages and crying spells. Connie feared that by expressing reactive anger, fear, and sadness after his death, she would appear to be too much like her mother.

4. *Information Processing: Prominent Ideas, Feelings, and Controls.* The death of her father set in motion a train of thought that would ideally define for her the meanings of her past relationships with him. Connie had important memories of idealized, happy times in his company. These were periods of apparently mutual admiration. But, after she sided with him, he became remote and soon married a woman much younger than himself. Connie interpreted his death as a final rejection, because it also included the impossibility of his ever reendorsing her worth.

She also felt as if his death was his way of punishing himself for rejecting her. That is, the early and unexpected stroke was seen as a psychosomatic response to his recognition that he had destroyed a meaningful attachment. When she began to experience resentment, however, she had to inhibit the ideas that incited this feeling, because anger caused her to feel too ashamed of being out of control and too guilty about hostility. If inhibition of ideas was insufficient, she tended to enter into altered states of consciousness such as the *distracted* state.

Process of Therapy

5. *States.* She had *intrusive crying* during the evaluation interview but warded off crying while talking with the therapist. The therapist detected her inhibition and blinking back of beginning tears. He told her that he would not feel critical of her if she did cry. She gradually became able to engage in *open crying*. As she worked through themes of mourning and of resentment toward her father, she was able to engage more and more of the time in a *working* state, expressing emotions with less feelings of being out of control.

Because the therapist was helpful and concerned, she could see him as an ideal father reestablishing the lost ideal relationship. During some episodes, she exhibited a *shining* state, which was like the one previously referred to as mutual admiration with her father. She also was occasionally skeptical and challenging of the therapist in mild trials to determine whether he could tolerate resentment.

Most of the time in therapy was spent by both persons working together. Early in therapy, however, there was a phase, repeated occasionally in later hours, in which she would begin each interview in the *distracted* state, not knowing what to say. This seemed to be a testing period, a therapeutic alliance was established, and *working* states ensued. There were periods of *sadness* in the concluding sessions.

6. *Relationship.* The therapeutic alliance seemed to be established right away because of her intense need. As her symptoms decreased rapidly over the first few sessions, however, Connie began to test the therapist to see if meaningful communication could take place. The critical issue was whether the therapist would see her as worthwhile or worthless because some of her attitudes might run counter to his presumed cultural stance of conformity and conservatism. These counter-cultural attitudes were also counterfather attitudes. As she found that the therapist did not refute or degrade her values, she herself tended to feel them as more authentic, and an increase in her self-esteem resulted. As self-esteem increased she was more willing to accept the challenge of further exploration of her ideas and feelings.

7. *Information Processing: Work on Ideas, Feelings, and Controls.* The main theme explored during therapy was the need to understand the meaning of her father's rejection of her. As the therapist began to counter some of her defensive inhibitions and denials, Connie was gradually able to get in touch with her resentment toward her father and her feelings of weakness and degradation. Emergence of her past history over the first series of sessions led to a gradual increase in focus on the present and future aspects of the therapy.

One of the important future themes interpreted by the therapist was Connie's tendency to repeat the relationship with her father in her selection of men whom she could idealize, but who were older, cold, and remote. It seemed that the death of her father also created a pivotal point at which she might reject men altogether, as persons who were incapable of returning love and care. Another version of this theme was the need to rescue men and some remorse that she had failed to rescue her father from what she saw as a psychosomatic illness.

Outcome

8. *States.* At the 3-month follow-up period she was no longer having episodes of *intrusive crying*. She was less depressed and felt generally more purposeful and able to have long periods in which she was in a *working* state.

9. Relationship. She felt an increased sense of self-worth. This was seen as a shift back to a position present before the father's death rather than a new development. At the follow-up she was still very much engaged in reviewing the meaning of her father's death and accepting the mourning process without fear or blocking. She was considering new relationships and had embarked on an attachment of unknown potential with a man.

10. Information Processing: Status of Ideas, Feelings, and Controls. The major change in the status of ideas was the development of a concept of the historical evolution and meaning of her relationship with her father. She integrated various self-images and relationship models so that she now had a central view of him not as cold and rejecting, but as presenting multiple self-images: as needing her while standing aloof and expressing an absence of need, as telling her to be independent while covertly telling her to be tied to his views and person. She was able to differentiate her fear of weakness, sadness at loss, resentment at scorn, and remoteness from "messy emotions," and also to develop a more complex, less stereotyped view of her mother. The premise that she could not feel angry with her father for being neurotically conflicted was altered so that she believed it acceptable to express anger with him and with related male figures. Because of these changes, she could allow herself to progress through waves of grief work characteristic of mourning. She was aware in part of her inhibitory operations, but no alteration of this style was noted.

STELLA: A SAMPLE REVIEW OF A PHENOMENON USING ONLY SOME STEPS

When a specific phenomenon is of interest, it can be reviewed using only the steps and points of view that seem most relevant. Specifying these steps gives boundaries to this discussion. In the following example, the phenomenon of interest was dissociated states and the process of splitting role relationship models. The temporal point of view covered the period of the therapy process. The conceptual points of view were state analysis (as in Chapters 2 and 5) and description of self-concepts and role relationship models (as in Chapters 3 and 6).

Identification

Stella was a young dentist who entered treatment during a state of general confusion precipitated by a disruptive love affair. This symptom subsided at once but treatment continued with a mutual goal of improvement of her capacity for work and interpersonal relationships. Developmentally, her character structure indicated that she had not formed a fully cohesive self-concept. Unlike the previous illustrative case, Stella was involved in extended rather than brief, time-limited psychoanalytic psychotherapy.

The period under consideration came after 1 year of treatment. During that time the actions of the therapist centered mainly on clarification and interpretation of her pattern of provocative and arrogant behavior toward colleagues. This behavior shielded her vulnerability to plummeting self-esteem but led to recurrent episodes of humiliation. During intensive work in centering attention on this pattern, Stella lost sight of why she was in psychotherapy. Although she did not contemplate quitting, she insisted upon challenging the therapist for an explanation of why she was still in treatment. The therapist summarized her pattern of provocative behavior with her colleagues and with him. She then rejected his concept of her as a person who sought help through treatment by reporting, to the surprise of the therapist, that for months she had told her colleagues that she was seeing the therapist as a form of special training to become a psychotherapist. The therapist's surprise was one of the reasons for selecting this episode for review.

It took some time for the therapist to realize that this story about being a trainee was not just provocation, arrogance, and acting out of a fantasy in the transference. For the moment, Stella actually believed what she had said, and had led others to believe that the therapist had asked her to be a special student. She used this explanation of her regular visits to justify them to her friends and, now, to herself.

The therapist tactfully confronted her with obvious evidence of the doctor-patient relationship and the defensive meaning of the special training theme. She reacted vehemently with brief episodes of righteous indignation and suspicion about his motives. She reviled and belittled him, accused him of instability, and of crazy projections. To support her arguments she drew upon her memory of what he had said at different times over the entire year, rearranging fragments to strengthen the special training theme. Gradually, over many hours, and during a painful struggle with grief and humiliation, she accepted her wish and need for treatment.

State Analysis

Stella segregated the meanings of being in therapy. In one state, to be called *mutuality A*, she knew quite well that she had come for treatment because of her behavior patterns and symptoms. She paid her fee for professional services and she worked for therapeutic changes in herself. But at times this placed her in a position of being a patient, of having impairments to a degree she could not tolerate. In another state, called *mutuality B*, she constructed a more agreeable alternative, using shreds of reality to see herself as a trainee. She **did** experiment with hypnosis as anesthesia in her dental practice. She **had** spent several weekends in encounter groups, and she **did** wish to be like the therapist. These concepts provided a scaffolding for the fantasy that the therapist had taken her into training as a lay therapist. Splitting, in terms of information processing, meant that she could organize everything the therapist had said as either his wish to teach her how to talk with patients or as his efforts as her therapist to help her with her problems. In either mutuality state, she related amiably with the therapist.

In the state marked by **righteous indignation**, Stella did not evaluate the training theme as fantasy. Instead, when confronted by the therapist with this idea, she regarded him as corrupt for having reneged on her training because of his lack of interest! During the working-through period, she oscillated between states of believing and not believing that she was a trainee. She could use brilliantly any remark or silence by the therapist to support either position. During interludes of her *mutuality* states, when she was cooperative and communicative, she made no mention of the occurrence of episodes of indignation and rage and seemed to ignore the therapist's references to such states, even if they had just occurred.

Two other states occurred during this period of therapy. One was *humiliation*, momentary because it was intolerably painful. The other state had an *aloof* characteristic. When in it, she was cold, arrogant, and distant. These will be described further in what follows.

Self-Images and Role Relationship Models

Stella had separate role relationship models. She processed specific events in terms of both constellations, but her appraisals from one set did not mitigate her appraisals in the other set. These recurrent role relationships, which were gradually defined as Stella shifted between states governed by them, are modeled in Figure 21.

The degree to which Stella was aware of only one state at a time, and the rapidity and fluidity of her change to an alternative state, was unusual. In this she resembled a borderline character typology (Kernberg, 1975). The four states modeled in this figure are those of the various role relationship models and self-concepts imposed by her on the treatment situation and on her current interpersonal relationships. There

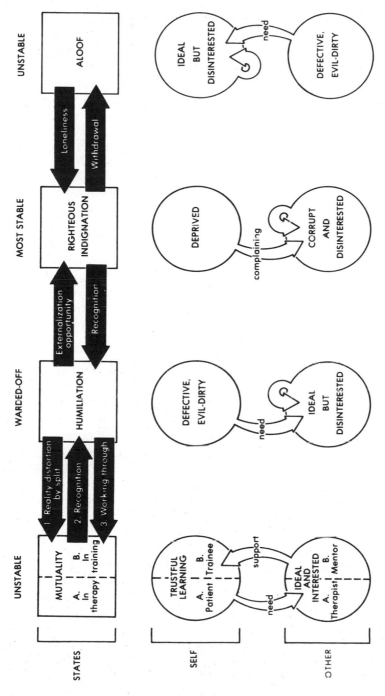

Figure 21. States and Underlying Role Relationships of Stella.

was, in addition, a realistic self-image and representation of the therapist, but this reality model was undependable and could not be maintained when she was in a state governed by the alternative schema.

Stella usually experienced the good or cooperative therapeutic condition, observed in the *mutuality A* state, as between a trustful learning child and an idealized and interested parent. Her fantasized ideal of being the therapist's trainee also fit this role model and, in the *mutuality B* state, stabilized a good self-image. With any stress on the therapeutic situation this role structure could not be maintained. In such crises of state change, she feared entry into the *humiliated* state where she would become a defective child, contaminated by evil, destructive, and dirty impulses. In this state, she felt unworthy of attention, and the parent image shifted from an ideal helper to one who was disinterested and distant. The searing feelings of humiliation and grief that resulted from this shift led her to avoid this state.

The threat of a shift from feeling good to feeling humiliated was related to two associative thoughts. If she was in the *mutuality A* state, representing herself as a patient, she could think of this as symbolic of defectiveness. The threat of being judged as defective made this state unstable. If she was in the *mutuality B* state, believing she was a trainee, she could think of being judged a fraud. This association could also evoke intense shame, making *mutuality B* also unstable. Being a patient was bad and true; being a trainee was good but untrue.

Instead of *humiliation*, the state most frequently enacted in the therapy was *righteous indignation*, where she felt and showed her rage at the therapist, whom she experienced as corrupt. She saw him as using therapy as a form of extortion, a way of taking excessive amounts of her money in return for very little, a put-on and a put-down. Another important recurrent episode was the *aloof* state. This state was based on a reversal of the self and other roles, from those of the feared and warded-off *humiliated* state. In the aloof state she experienced the therapist as a needy, defective, dirty person, in relation to herself as totally sufficient. He could attempt pathetically weak and inadequate remarks as she watched, remote, disdainful, and without response.

The change between these states followed observable patterns in the therapy, in her reports of everyday life, and in her memories and fantasies of childhood. She liked and attempted to maintain the *mutuality* states. But clarifications, interpretations, and the insults of everyday life seemed like criticisms that destroyed this fragile balance and threatened to precipitate the *humiliated* state. To ward off emergence or continuance of this *humiliated* state, she shifted her self and object model to that of either the *righteous indignation* or *aloof* states.

To emphasize this point, she can be described as having split apart rather than integrated schemata of self and other. Usually the shift from the role models of the *mutuality* states to those of the *humiliated* state was not defensive but can be seen in terms of process, as a failure of capacity for regulation, and in terms of structure, as a developmental arrest in that she was unable to maintain a coherent, stable self-image in the face of personal blemishes. The *humiliated* state was so painful that she would then defend herself against it by resorting to the self-images and roles of the *righteous indignation* or *aloof* states. For her, *righteous indignation* was a relatively sturdy position. Once stabilized in it she might regain the *mutuality A* state either because her anger provoked the other person to increased support or because she was able to make a progressive move. If she felt respected by the therapist she could regain *mutuality A*; if she saw herself as in training she could regain *mutuality B*. From a temporary stance in the *aloof* state she had to move to the state of *righteous indignation* because she could not stand loneliness, or to the *mutuality* states when she needed to restore her self-esteem.

To provide a nidus of reality, Stella provoked others to behave in a way that fitted a given alternate relationship model. Her most frequent manipulation involved behaving in such a way that roles were reversed, as in her shift from *righteous indignation* to the *aloof* state.

Working Through Ideas about Self-Images and Relationship Models during Therapy

There was a period of working through in which Stella knew what was coming next in therapy. She knew that the therapist would repeat the statement that she was not a special trainee if she went on as if this was what she believed. She also sensed that she could exasperate the therapist by continuing to tell this story to others. He might be embarrassed by a situation where others would think that instead of conducting treatment he had taken an attractive young woman under his wing in an unauthorized and corrupt training program. If she delayed recognizing the fantasy nature of the special training image, the therapist would be provoked into repeating that she was not a trainee. Not only would this comment hurt her feelings, but the form might be too firm, too exasperated, or too harsh. Even if he were silent, the therapist could be seen as either neglectful or as confirming the mildly delusional belief. The therapist had to tactfully tiptoe along this fine line and Stella watched him do so. Indeed, both parties watched and it was now the therapist who could make mistakes.

This type of externalization of roles had therapeutic aspects. Stella could here make the therapeutic split into what has been called the observing and the experiencing ego (Greenson, 1967). But it was the therapist who was observed as he acted out the part she gave him. In the *aloof* state she viewed the therapist as acting the role of a defective, dirty, evil, aggressive person. But in a detached way she also observed how he handled situations in which he was provoked to assume this role. She learned how he handled the provocation, controlled himself, and maintained his calm. By modeling herself on what she observed, she learned both to avoid the *humiliated* state and to tolerate its threatening self-images. In other words, she learned by identification with the therapist how to handle and tolerate her own most feared position (Loewald, 1960).

This vignette has provided a condensed application of configurational analysis to a difficult clinical phenomenon. The explanation was a partial one. A fuller explanation would involve examining additional points of view and articulating them with the patterns described. The developmental reasons for her present character structure could be postulated. Her other problems and behavior patterns could be related to the explanations already advanced. **For teaching purposes, such idealized or "complete" explanations are usually too time-consuming. They may also be too difficult when the undertaking leads into areas where insufficient or unclear data are all that are available. But any attempt to link observations to explanatory theories is useful. Some aspects of the configurational analysis approach can be used according to what seems most relevant to understanding a given context.** In the above example, the primary focus was on structural characteristics, the different inner models of self and role relationship. In the following example, the primary focus, again using only some steps of configurational analysis, is on information-processing issues.

THE SECOND EXAMPLE: INFORMATION-PROCESSING STYLE

In the next teaching example, another behavioral pattern and another dramatic episode in therapy were noted and used as the focus for explanatory effort. The pattern consisted of a general style in which the patient expressed information to the therapist and proceeded to assimilate that information. The single dramatic episode was one in which the patient's state changed in the therapy and he composed a short poem symbolic of ideas that were difficult to assimilate. The task set for a limited configurational analysis was to understand the function of this special episode, the processing of information, the conscious and nonconscious sets of ideas during different phases of the treatment hour.

Ronald, a graduate student in his late 20s, lived as an intellectual hermit. Although he was brilliant, he was socially immature and professionally unsuccessful. "Narcissistic personality disorder" would be the closest diagnosis. The episode of interest occurred during the second year of psychoanalytic psychotherapy.

Ronald's style of expression and assimilation in therapy was as follows. He characteristically brought in an emotionally toned current experience. He did not know clearly what the emotions were or why the experience bothered him. Implicitly, he expected that he and the therapist would explore this together. They would then "find out" that the experience gave rise to ideas that wounded his self-esteem and caused sadness, fear, humiliation, anger, or self-disgust. He would then parade the negative emotion in an exhibitionistic way, enjoying this activity as a sign of his successful work in treatment and as evidence of the therapist's attention and "gifts of insight." As will be seen, this form of interpersonal relationship paralleled the content of the warded-off ideas and feelings.

In previous hours Ronald had worked sporadically—to a degree that was tolerable for him—on his fear of the various rituals of sexual courtship. When he was forward in caressing a woman, he felt endangered by a humiliating rejection. When he was passive with a woman, he feared being labeled as not virile. He commonly assumed a pose of arrogant nonchalance to maintain poise and self-esteem.

He began the hour in question by talking about the previous evening spent with a woman friend. He was characteristically nonchalant as he mentioned the important fact, almost as an aside, that he had engaged in intercourse with her for the first time. The incident he brought in for this hour was that he had noticed that "something haunted him about the occasion." This incident occurred a moment prior to intercourse. They had undressed some feet apart from each other and he had seen her glancing at him. Ronald recalled thinking of himself, "I have a handsome and tanned head but my body must look old because it is white and soft."

After telling of the haunting quality of the memory, of the glance, and his idea of a young head on an old body, he then entered a *reverie* state, which was his self-centered version of free association. It is described as self-centered because there was reason to believe that he experienced it with a self-image like that of a child asleep and dreaming, perceiving the therapist, only remotely, as a kind of parent, or guardian angel who watched over him. In a manner similar to Kohut's (1971, 1977) description of the idealizing mirror transference, Ronald had no sense of the therapist as a cohesive person during this experience but saw him more as a kind of two-dimensional "guardian." He also seemed to have little or no sense of reflective self-awareness (Schafer, 1968).

In this *reverie* state, he processed information in an experiential mode. That is, he reexperienced the incident with the woman through a revisualization of the scene. He described again the idea of his body being old and his head young. He made the association of "old" as "unattractive"; he supposed the woman might find his white body old and unattractive.

Warded-Off Ideas

The ideational constellation can now be described. Some emergent contents were inhibited because they threatened to cause excessive emotional pain if they were directly and clearly experienced. These ideas emerged gradually into consciously experienced thoughts during the hour.

The conscious ideas, "My body is white," and the implied idea, "She may find it unattractive," tended to evoke the respondent idea, "My body will really age." This is outlined in Figure 22.

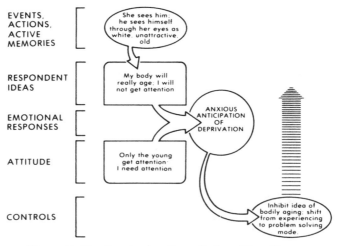

Figure 22. The Deprivation Constellation of Ronald.

The respondent idea, "My body will really age," was inhibited from conscious representation because it led to anxiety, since it matched associatively with an enduring attitude, "Only the young get attention," an attitude based in turn on oedipal memories and fantasies. The memory was of his success in diverting his mother's attention from his father, who was old. The fantasy was developed according to the Talion principle that punishment for replacing his father was to age as his father had aged. There was also a plausible preoedipal configuration, although there was insufficient evidence to be certain of this. According to Ronald, his mother stopped treating him as "his majesty the baby" as he grew from infancy to childhood, and instead indulged a younger sibling, while he felt neglected.

The associational match led to another respondent idea, that he would not get attention. Not getting attention did not mesh well with an enduring but warded-off attitude of needing continuous attention from others. The threat of experiencing such thoughts in conscious form generated anxious anticipation of the loss of love and self-stability. The composite emotional experience would be potentially intolerable if inhibitory controls did not prevent conscious representation of these ideas.

Information Processing and Change in Controls

Let us return now to the stream of experience described by Ronald during the hour. He was in a state of thinking the conscious ideas and warding off the respondent ideas diagrammed in Figure 22. His capacity to totally inhibit the "My body will really age" idea was inadequate to the emergent power of this association. He experienced this idea consciously but then disavowed its import by a series of control maneuvers that accomplished two aims: They diluted his conscious emotional experience to a tolerable dose, and they eventually led to a clear and conscious expression of the once warded-off ideas.

The first noticeable maneuver was to change the concrete personal image of the woman looking at him, and even the less object-oriented idea of his body aging, to an abstract principle: not "My body will age" or "My body is older," but "Bodies age." Concomitantly, he shifted his thought organization from an experiential mode (experiencing his associational responses) to a problem-solving mode. That is, he changed to an *analytic* state in which he was thinking of implications and possible recombinations of associations in order to achieve a specific goal. His particular problem-solving mode was the formulation of a poem. Poetic form of a certain type was familiar to him; he liked to compose haiku.

The organizing structure of these poems is to juxtapose two evocative contrasting ideas to arrive at a third line that synthesizes them both.

In this problem-solving mode he therefore had a predetermined and automatized plan: to take the idea "Bodies age," find a potentially related but contrasting idea to juxtapose, and then show the connection between the two ideas. This switch from responding in an experiential mode to operating in a problem-solving mode temporarily halted the ideational cycle of linear associations that would lead to representation of the warded-off contents (Klein, 1967). Instead, he now "knew" what else to think: If "Bodies age" represented a loss, he had to think of a relevant gain. He selected sensibility, a kind of wisdom of the mind, as the benefit of aging. The loss (attractiveness) and gain (sensibility-wisdom) juxtaposed well with the poignant, bittersweet, evocative quality of the short poem. (The three ideas were "Bodies age," "One gains sensibility-wisdom with time," and "The second compensates for the first.") The poem "read" well and he felt a thrill imagining an audience's response. There was, again, a narcissistic gain to compensate for a narcissistic loss.

While it is not possible to report the actual poem, a similar substitute has been contrived. Although it is not as aesthetically pleasing as the original, it conveys the ideational movement with symbolic similarity.

Old hawk wings droop with time yet hover still
Sharply sudden the deft swoop through needle's eye
How expertly this ancient warrior pierces his target prey

As he imagined the audience or reader response, Ronald switched from the *analytic* state of problem solving, presenting ideas in the form of a haiku, back to the *reverie* state. During this state and its experiential mode of thinking he fantasized how someone else would respond emotionally to his poem. In the context of this return to the experiential mode, he then experienced anxiety and sadness in an attenuated form, as poignancy that was tolerable because something was gained as well as something lost. This emotional experience was not clearly located; it was neither in himself nor in his imagined audience but somehow included both. There was, however, a relative reversal of self-image, from a passive role to an active one. He then switched back from the *reverie* state to the *analytic* state. This change in state occurred as he became aware of the relationship between himself and the therapist. In this *analytic* state he reflected on the therapist's responses to the poem, which will be described after a brief summary of matters thus far.

Ronald diluted a gradual emergence and experience of warded-off mental contents by a series of cognitive maneuvers. These maneuvers involved (1) inhibition of representation of the warded-off contents; (2) change from a personal, concrete instance to an abstract concept; (3) change from an experiential mode (allowing responsive associations) to a problem-solving mode (composing a poem); (4) decrease in reflective self-awareness and increase in awareness of the presence of the therapist; and (5) associations of the therapist's possible responses to the haiku and to ideas of the therapist as aging.

Working Through Warded-Off Ideas and Feelings

As he thought of the therapist's response, Ronald decided that the therapist was old and therefore "whiter" and "softer" than he, but that maybe the therapist could tolerate this because he had accumulated wisdom. This externalization allowed him to contemplate the warded-off ideas and feelings and appraise the degree of threat through identification with the therapist. Could the therapist stand it? From this point of view, the construction of esthetic symbols or "names" aids contemplation of emotion rather than intense and direct experiencing of emotional states (Langer, 1942).

Deciding that the therapist was all right (that is, not too threatened by either the thrust of his powerful creative achievement or by their comparative ages), Ronald switched from the *analytic* state (thinking of what went on between them) to the experiential state of associative *reverie*. He developed associations clustered around his enduring attitude that only the young can get attention, and getting older pushes you "offstage." There was then a brief negation of the topic—he was not old but young—and another return to the hard-to-accept ideas that he too would really age. There were then switches from the *reverie* state to the *analytic* state ("What would the therapist think of his associations?"— his version at this point of a self-observing function) and back to *reverie* with further associations that led eventually to his conscious experience of the warded-off contents.

Toward the end of the hour, then, he had the capacity to think and feel contents that had been warded off earlier in the hour. His shift to poetry writing allowed a period of what could summarily be called denial, although it was actually a composite of defensive maneuvers. During this period he progressively assimilated threatening ideas and feelings. The poetry writing in particular, entailed a switch away from the experiential mode, an alteration in self-object attitudes, and a wishful, narcissistic compensation for a threatened blow to his self-esteem.

At the end of the hour Ronald stood up and announced that he would write down the poem and that he had "really gotten something" from the hour. This savoring of "getting" and his capacity to compose the poem reassured him; he had a safe retreat. In a way, he could tolerate the threat of the warded-off ideas, and the relationship with the therapist could be reviewed and yet denied, a way station on the path to integration and acceptance.

What was worked through here were some previously warded-off ideas and feelings about a particular life event, as related past experiences were allowed representation, and the event was assimilated. His style of avoiding threatening ideas and feelings was not altered by the one hour, but repetition of such work gradually increased his tolerance for painful ideas, cut down generalizations based on childhood experience, and reduced the extensiveness and intensiveness of his unconscious defensive operations. His defensive style, narcissistic vulnerability, and enduring attitudes were chipped away, not worked through. As for the transference situation, this hour was a repetition. Once again he paraded a "discovered" negative emotion in an exhibitionistic way. The transference evolved a little, and together with realistic goals of self-awareness, motivated the working through of the stressful life event. But Ronald gained no insight into the transference aspects of this hour, and they were not interpreted at this time in the treatment.

The Case Fragment in the Larger Context of the Therapeutic Process

The above discussion focused on information processing in a single hour. If it were a fully developed case report, the focus would have been on longer-order patterns of relationship, such as the patient's use of an idealizing transference to bolster an impairment in maintaining a cohesive self-concept. The reader may tend to enlarge on the small-order patterns in order to imagine the large-order patterns involved in the patient's character pathology and may wonder what interpretations were involved in the treatment. As stated, no interpretations were made by the therapist in this particular hour. The therapist operated as a presence—only partially experienced by the patient, but nonetheless a presence—who occasionally (like a rudder) suggested quite minor adjustments that kept the patient safely on a course. These few comments on the treatment are made only to clarify what is not under discussion here, the relationship issues of transference, resistance to transference, interpretation of transference, and genesis.

Interpretive activity did precede and follow the hour. Alone, Ronald would not have extended the meanings of the stressful event because the emotional threat (anxiety and/or humiliation) was too great. In the therapeutic relationship, the emotional threat was reduced, and the anticipation of transference gratification motivated an elaboration of ideas and feelings that were usually warded off. Interpretations of resistance and fears about intimacy, trust, and self-exposure had preceded this moment in therapy. Such work led to the existing alliance, the protective umbrella of relationship that allowed the patient to work out his ideas without immediate interpretation.

During the hour reported the therapist did not interpret meanings of the material that were too threatening. The patient's sense of self-esteem and safety was enhanced by his own capacity to work out the event and its significance. In subsequent hours it was possible to return to the memorable product, the poem, and elaborate further meanings. Some of these relationship models can now be briefly mentioned.

The episode of intercourse was a major stress as well as an accomplishment. The patient's anxieties about sex and performance were as important as, or more important than, his worries about his appearance. He was afraid of being judged inferior, and the hawk and prey dyad of the poem was symbolic of a particular self- and object schema. One role was that of a strong, sadistic aggressor, the other of a helpless, faceless, or amorphous prey.

The poem was a wish fulfillment. It posited him as the hawk, the woman as prey. He was capable of "piercing" fully and was not in danger of impotence. The self-object dyad was a reversal of the most fearful version of the same schema, in which he was the characterless prey. The clarification of this aspect of the episode, as well as certain sadistic aspects of his sexuality, required subsequent interpretation and much more extended working through.

SUMMARY

The overall format of configurational analysis, and the methods used to help the process of observation, analysis, and description of each step are useful in helping trainees to understand processes of change. A complete configurational analysis can be time-consuming if all ten steps are followed in detail. But any case will have some particular features. One step or several steps of configurational analysis most suitable to a selected focus can be executed, with an open-ended understanding that additional levels of explanation are possible. This partial task is less time-consuming and therefore more practical when case review must be a limited effort.

Configurational analysis can be done from process notes, case summaries, or recordings. It is possible for training centers to build a library containing a variety of completed cases. Trainees can then take the raw data and attempt any of the configurational analysis steps, in any degree of detail. They can then compare their results with those of others. When disagreements in inference are found, they can return to the basic data in search of further observations that will support one or another point of view. In this way, the empirical and observational basis of theory will become apparent to them or, better yet, their work will revise theory so that it conforms more closely to what can be observed.

CHAPTER TWELVE

Research Applications
with Nancy Wilner and Charles Marmar

In each step of configurational analysis assertions are made about patterns that characterize the person in a specific context. Once these statements are clear, it is possible to check their reliability using information retained by recording or notation and thus available to review. Reliability of the configurational analysis method rests with the degree to which a second or third person, blind to the pattern judgments of the first reviewer, can follow the same system and produce comparable results.

When independent clinicians review process notes, audiotapes, or videotapes, they share instructions and guidelines. Their task is to observe the data, describe the patterns, and fit the contents to the given format. Their independent assertions are compared for similarities and differences. What is agreed upon can be set aside. What remains are differences to be further discussed so that semantic confusions are resolved and separated from substantial disparity. Residual differences can then be formulated to the point of operational definition of observations that would support or undermine each position. The data can then be reviewed again from the point of view of these operational definitions. Through such a process **differences are seen not only as evidence of unreliability, but as indications of areas in need of closer observation, sharper classification, and clearer theoretical formulation.**

Any step that seems particularly decisive for a given patient can serve as the beginning for such studies. If no particular step seems pertinent, then state-judgments serve as a good beginning. They are closest to observation, and a pivotal point for later elaborations. Independent observers can then use the various states to describe the self-images and role relationships that correlate with them. This would follow the method mentioned above of working independently with the same data and then comparing results. Once a state list is agreed upon, the next question concerns whether judges can concur upon a given moment as an instance of a particular state.

The following illustrative research was conducted with the case of Janice, using the state descriptions listed in Chapter 2.

Illustration: The Reliability of State Descriptions. The first step to test the reliability of state descriptions was to have two additional judges (N.W. and C.M.) review videotapes of interviews to determine their degree of agreement with the initial descriptions. These judges worked together, finding discussions beneficial in sharpening observation, and thus developed their own descriptions for each state. The original state names were acceptable and were used as the basic labels for the major states. The descriptive format was elaborated by the two judges into three subcategories for listing patterns of states: behavioral form, verbal content, and degree of congruity between form and content. Some of the state descriptions from Chapter 2 (Table 4) are repeated here for convenience in Table 20A, and the expanded descriptions by the two judges are added in Table 20B. For the ensuing tests these judges used their own operational definitions (Table 20B).

The next procedure was aimed at determining whether the two judges, operating independently, could agree on specific material as representing a particular state. To avoid scoring very momentary shifts, a state was operationally defined as lasting for at least 10 seconds before it could be scored. Thirty-six 10-minute segments from the 6 odd-numbered treatment hours were ordered according to a table of random numbers, and the first four 10-minute segments of videorecorded material were selected, with the stipulation that no two segments from the same hour would be used. The resulting 40-minute test material contained 10-minute segments from hours 3, 1, 11, and 7, in that order. Judges synchronized their stopwatches, marked the time of each transition of state, and named the new states entered at these points.

In the interest of accuracy, judges viewed each 10-minute tape segment a second time immediately after the first viewing, in order to make any additions or corrections that they thought were indicated. Only then did they compare results. An agreement was defined by stringent conditions; that is, the timing had to be the same, predefined as plus or minus 7.5 seconds, and the state said to be entered had also to be the same. If either judge scored a change, the other judge had to be rated as agreeing or disagreeing.

There was a range of 11 to 18 state transitions judged for each 10-minute segment, making for a total of over 68 points for agreement or disagreement. The agreement rate was 73%.

Table 20A. Detailed Observations about Recurrent States

Main states during therapy

1. *Tra-la-la*—engaging, perky, histrionic, gestures are wide and outward, attention on other, smiles, makes faces, fast-talking, interrupts. Pretends to feel but is distant from the stated ideas. May play-act or exaggerate her own ideas and feelings while feeling inwardly at a distance from them. Would like to feel mutually engaged with another, or actively creative, but feels inwardly at a distance from these ideals as well.

2. *Hurt but working*—head down, shamed or depressed; holding, rubbing, or picking self with hands, more leaden face, talks more slowly and softly; reflective on self, attention inward.

Other states

3. *Hurt and not working*—withdrawn, reads, overeats, refuses social invitations, mumbles and trails off during interview; feels foggy and unreal; depressed, has bodily concerns, sad, lonely.

4. *Competitive/angry*—critical of or struggling with others to see who will control or dominate the situation, who is to blame if it doesn't go well; edge in voice, feels contempt, indignation, or anger; challenges other to prove worth; can escalate to temper outburst.

5. *Acute self-disgust*, shame, or despair—feels revulsion at being fat, unaccomplished; self-critical, inactive, withdrawn, silly, pretending, or sexually wrong (too active, too inactive). Most other states are to ward off this one.

Table 20B. State Descriptions as Elaborated by Two Judges

Definition of terms:	Behavioral form:	Posture, facial expression, tone of voice, gestures, flow of speech, deployment of attention
	Verbal content:	Reports of thoughts, feelings, behaviors
	Congruence-incongruence:	Degree of synergy between form and content

1. *Tra-la-la*

Behavioral form:

Engaging, perky, histrionic verbalization and gestures, deployment of attention on others, smiles, makes faces, speaks quickly, interrupts, raises voice, gestures outward, sits forward, highly animated.

Verbal content:

Often angry, competitive, flirtatious, uses mimicry to express hostile, contemptuous feelings, singsong quality to voice; variant to this is social chitchat, with lessening of dramatic quality and appearance of mutality, lacking in authenticity; failure to recognize own feelings (especially hostility).

(Continued)

Table 20B. (*Continued*)

1. *Tra-la-la* (*continued*)	
Incongruence:	Play-acts or exaggerates ideals and feelings while being at a distance from them, pretends, wishes to feel mutually engaged and actively creative, but is inwardly at a distance from these ideals.
2. *Hurt but working*	
Behavioral form:	Head down, holds hands together, rubs and picks at self, slow soft speech, sad or hurt look, attention turned inward, bodily stillness.
Verbal content:	Reflective comments on self, comments or thoughts turned inward, analytic about self and others. Communicates thoughts and feelings authentically and with self-awareness.
Congruence:	Form and content express self-examination, painful work.
3. *Hurt and not working*	
Behavioral form:	Withdrawn, attention directed inward, may throw head back or downward in despair, speaks slowly, mumbles, trails off.
Verbal content:	Comments reflecting hopelessness, demoralization, sadness, loneliness, depression. Reports feeling foggy and unreal. Expresses bodily concerns. Does not have access to information available in other states.
Congruence:	Form and content express and demonstrate hopelessness.
4. *Competitive-angry*	
Behavioral form:	Attention directed outward to involve other. Challenging or contemptuous edge to voice, which may be raised, usually with increased flow of speech. Occasional pounding of chair arm, direct eye contact, chin out, arms occasionally extended.
Verbal content:	Struggle for control of situation, challenging and critical of the worth of others, concern with blame, expresses feelings of contempt, indignation, anger. Can escalate to temper outburst.
Congruence:	Expresses and demonstrates competitiveness and hostility.
5. *Acute self-disgust*	
Behavioral form:	Looks away, lowers voice, half smiles, speaks slowly, plays with hair, raises eyebrows, repeats key word several times (demand, suck, give me).
Verbal content:	Feelings of self-contempt, self-hatred, shame, guilt, negative body image (fat, ugly, hairy), passivity, defective feminine self-image, unaccomplished. Aware of defects and tends to exaggerate them.
Congruence:	Experiences and communicates self-disgust.

Table 21. Frequency of Agreement on Judgment of States and State Transitions (Mean of Two Judges) on a Sample of Four 10-Minute Segments[a]

State entered	Mean episodes	Mean duration of episodes (and range) in seconds	Mean % agreement
Tra-la-la	24	42 (10–175)	74%
Hurt but working	28	35 (10–120)	74%
Hurt and not working	4	28 (10–55)	83%
Competitive/angry	4	22 (10–40)	46%
Self-disgust	2	23 (15–30)	83%
Summary	Total = 62	Mean = 30 (10–175)	Mean = 73%

[a]From Horowitz, Marmar, and Wilner (1979).

As shown in Table 21, the most frequent and also the longest episodes (as stated in Chapters 2 and 5) were the *tra-la-la* and *hurt but working* states.

Operating independently, these judges achieved good reliability. In discussion of differences, it was clear that even better reliability could be achieved by jointly viewing videotaped segments, discussing observations, repeating the basic data, and then making either agreed-upon or disagreed-upon judgments. For these reasons, the ensuing work was conducted by both judges working together.

The next problem was the examination of states to determine if there was empirical evidence for the descriptive statement by the author in Chapter 5 that certain states changed in frequency during therapy. The data for these analyses were other segments of video-recordings. A 10-minute segment from minute 30 to minute 40 was taken from each of the 12 therapy hours. This time period was selected on theoretical grounds as a representative segment because it avoided the beginning and end of treatment hours, when issues of settling down to work and arrangements for future meetings are commonplace, and focused on an expectably productive section of the hour. The segments were arranged by a technician according to a table of random numbers, and judges did not know which hour they reviewed as they made their judgments. (Estimates of which hour they saw were inaccurate.) These judgments, as before, determined when a state transition occurred, and labeled the state that was entered.

As mentioned earlier, the major states during the therapy hours were the *hurt but working* and *tra-la-la* states. The other states occurred but were less frequent and briefer in duration. As predicted, the *tra-la-la* state was most prominent in the early hours and declined over the 12 hours of therapy. Increasingly more time was spent in the *hurt but working* state as therapy progressed. The pattern of these data is shown in Figure 23.

In Chapter 5, phases of therapy were described in relation to state changes. Those assertions were written before this quantitative approach to the data was undertaken. Phase one comprised the first 2 hours; the assertion was that Janice was mostly in the *tra-la-la* state. This hypothetical pattern was found in the quantitative study as indicated by the graph of Figure 23. In the second phase, hours 3 and 4, the *hurt but working* state was said to emerge more clearly. This assertion was also supported by the two judges with their quantitative measure of state lengths.

A third phase was earlier delineated as hours 5, 6, and 7. This phase was described as containing transitions between the two main states that occurred to test the therapist with evidence of a growing relationship between therapist and patient. As shown in Figure 23, the decline of *tra-la-la* and the reciprocal increase of the *hurt but working* state in these 3 hours attest to this relationship. During the remaining hours, the primary ideational work of the therapy was said to occur in a fairly stable therapeutic alliance. This is reflected by the low frequency of the *tra-la-la* state found in the quantitative analysis of these hours.

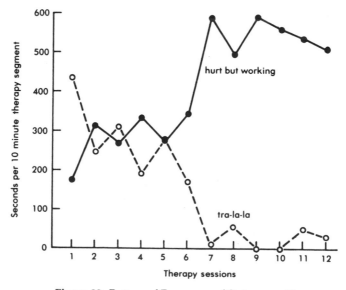

Figure 23. Pattern of Frequency of States over Time.

To recapitulate, such quantitative studies as these (Marmar, Wilner, and Horowitz, 1984) can be extended to examine the reliability of the assertions advanced, using the configurational analysis method. Once states can be judged, as shown above, it would be possible to assemble segments of a recorded therapy according to the more important states described for that person. Then the data for each state could be examined and compared with other states by content analysis (or ratings) of self-images, role models, communicative interactions, or particular styles of control and defense. Any hypotheses of particularly prominent patterns of state shifts as instigated by therapist actions could also be checked for reliability and for size of effect by similar quantitative means.

APPLICATIONS IN CLINICAL INVESTIGATION

The two most important paths toward variations in patterns would apply the method to different types of persons and to different schools of therapy. Well-known types such as the histrionic and obsessional personalities may change in different ways. They may elicit different types of therapist behavior. Even the nuances of clarification and interpretation may be carried out differently by the therapist with different types of persons. It would be useful to compare change processes in a number of persons with hysterical personality to observe similarities and differences, and to highlight them by contrasts with change processes abstracted from a group of obsessional patients. Clinical investigations do this all the time, but the steps of configurational analysis could sharpen the process by providing a systematic format.

The second path examines change processes that result from different tactics of intervention. Many schools of therapy exist, but it is unlikely that processes of change are divided according to such boundaries. Interventions explained by the therapist according to one theoretical system may work effectively for other reasons.

A useful research approach would involve retaining data from various kinds of therapy, reviewing these data by the methods described here, and so assembling a theory of different, albeit interactive, processes of change. A focus on controls is central to this endeavor since most therapies act to alter the patient's current level and manner of self-regulation. Some techniques make controls less necessary by supplying external controls or safe situations. Others force the patient to set aside controls because of social pressure. State changes certainly occur in both kinds of therapy. But what structural changes occur and remain? And with what kind of person, in terms of habitual control styles? As already mentioned, such research will develop more extensive formats for use in configurational analysis. It will also clarify general issues across schools of therapy, moving toward a general psychology of change processes.

Articulation with Quantitative Data

Configurational analysis can articulate numerical data from groups of clinical research patients and give qualitative meanings. Suppose that a clinical population has been given a treatment procedure. Outcome evaluations will show a range of improvement that spans the least to the most improved. The range of outcome scores on rating scales will indicate the position of various individuals, but these scores will not explain why the patient is in this position or relate it to other factors. If hypotheses were formulated one could do correlational analyses between variables, but such hypotheses must be generated with clarity before such quantitative studies can be conducted. Configurational analysis can be used to develop such hypotheses and explore variables too complexly interactive for simple correlations.

As a start, one may compare individuals with similar characteristics who fared well, with those who did not. Hypotheses generated by such work can be clarified further by selecting additional cases along the range of outcomes. After explanatory principles are fairly clear, content analyses or new rating scales could be used to seek correlational tests of suspected relationships. Or, if a treatment program were ongoing, and if findings suggested changes in treatment strategy, then such changes could be instituted conducting forward regression analyses of outcome levels to see if effectiveness of treatment increased. If group comparisons were possible, more decisive tests of hypothetically active change agents could be conducted using control groups to contrast with populations who receive that treatment.

Configurational analysis can be used with representative cases from the different groups even in such control group designs. Suppose that two kinds of treatment were offered to drug-dependent persons: Group A was detoxified and released; Group B was placed on maintenance drug substitution. Or, suppose that a group of persons with acute anxiety disorders were offered brief psychoanalytically oriented psychotherapy and a comparable group was offered therapy with a newer technique. Standard statistical comparisons would be done on quantitative data derived from scales. On such analyses one would find a range of responses to both Treatment A and Treatment B. Many subjects from each group might benefit, and some subjects from each group might suffer apparent harm (Strupp, Hadley, and Gomes-Schwartz, 1977). Comparisons of group means show only which treatment was "better." But if only a few cases were harmed, quantitative explanation or understanding of the processes involved would be unlikely. Again, one can select individual cases for careful study by configurational analysis. Work on such individual cases allows more extensive interpretation of the quantitative data, especially since the position of the individual in relation to the group is already known. (For an example, see Horowitz, Marmar, Krupnick, *et al.*, 1984).

The Development of Typologies

Repetition of configurational analysis with subjects from a large group can lead to clusters of persons who resemble each other in defined ways. The usual manner of classifying or typologizing persons is by their problems or observed maladaptive behavior. Another method is to find typologies by state lists as described in Chapter 2. As state lists are assembled for each person, repetitions will be noted, and determinations of the underlying self-images and role relationships will be made. A cluster of persons may emerge from this analysis who seem quite similar, at least in terms of their manifestation of a given state and the coherence of their self-concept and role relationship models within that state.

The Axis 2 Disorders of DSM-III and the classical psychoanalytic typologies of hysterical, obsessional and borderline characters (Salzman, 1968; Horowitz, 1977a; Kernberg, 1975) are in effect such configurationally defined typologies. That is, the classical type will tend to have certain relatively specific problems in times of stress and even be relatively vulnerable to certain types of stress. They will tend to have their own kind of states and state transitions. They will have their own problematic role relationship and self-image constellations. They will be similar in information-processing style as seen by their tendency to certain affective responses to specific types of ideational conflicts and their habitual use of particular defenses.

The definition of typologies requires consensual validation by many clinicians. **But when many clinicians write about a character style, their statements seldom follow any order and usually focus primarily on one particular aspect. Configurational analysis provides a format for such work on defining typologies.**

SUMMARY

Dynamic psychology has been criticized for its vagueness of theory and for the unreliability of its observations. Moreover, even when theories have been clearly stated, the evidence that might refute or confirm the theory has been alluded to vaguely but not described. When observations are presented, they have been described as biased, and based on inadequate sampling. Configurational analysis as a research method may supply a way of linking observations to theory and so answer such criticisms.

Configurational analysis is a method for individual pattern description. It aims to clarify the state, structure, and process that characterize a period of change in the life of a person. As many different individuals are studied by configurational analysis, repetitions of patterns will be found. Just as personality typologies have gradually evolved from this sort of description, it may now be possible to describe typologies of change process. While the precursory theories are based on psychoanalytic, information-processing, and learning theory, the basic psychology of configurational analysis is general enough to allow study of any intervention strategy. Using such an approach, it should be possible to examine the processes that help and harm patients treated by various schools of psychotherapy.

To advance the method of configurational analysis itself, further applications to test and increase reliability and expand formats are indicated. As the method evolves, it can fill the gap between what is known from quantitative therapy research and what is observed from clinical vignettes based on skilled observation, with periodic use of clinical judges and quantitative methods.

CHAPTER THIRTEEN

Applications during Treatment

While the use of configurational analysis enhances teaching and extends theory, it may also have direct application in treatment settings. The therapist, alone or in consultation, may use this method as an aid to formulation and goal setting early in therapy. It also provides a practical method for reviewing the situation and revising intervention tactics during periods of impasse. It can be utilized selectively as a technique when increased insight into patterns such as state cycles might help a patient implement more adaptive controls.

UTILIZATION FOR THE WORKING MODELS OF THE THERAPIST

Empathy and intuitive response are valuable, possibly essential ingredients in psychotherapy. The intellectual effort of configurational analysis is not contrary to such skills; it can heighten them. Intuition is rapid information processing involving no conscious recognition and memory for sequential steps in the formation of a concept. Intellectual processing is slower, more conscious, and deliberate. **Intuition is usually necessary in the conduct of psychotherapy because so much is happening so rapidly, in a multilayered matrix, that the therapist can never hope to examine intellectually any but the most relevant information. Intellectual review is possible only when the time pressures of active therapy are absent, when contemplation can occur without the necessity for immediate responsivity. Then intuitive working models, fragmentary hunches, and important but incompletely appraised observations can be reworked according to the steps of configurational analysis. Done at some point during treatment, such reviews prepare the mind**

so that intuition can then operate during the therapy hour itself facilitating focused expectation, rapid appraisals, and comprehensive pattern recognition.

The intellectual tasks of configurational analysis can be performed
by the therapist after a few initial visits. This task, done in a general
way, may not be complete but can prepare the mind of the therapist for
new observations. To the extent that it is completed, models of relationship issues may aid the therapist in predicting potential tests for
transference possibilities or for avoidance of social relationship in the
therapeutic work. Challenges can be anticipated and plans made to
handle them. From constellations of ideas, feelings, and controls, the
therapist develops working models of themes that are uppermost, and
of pitfalls to be avoided, and will have a chance for preliminary thoughts
on difficulties and potential routes to solution. The interrelationships
between habitual information processing (or avoiding) styles and various
self-images, relationship models, and potential states can be explored,
preparing the therapist for possibly decisive moments.

This method is also useful as a review when the therapist has a
sense that the treatment process is at an impasse or stalemated by a
covert, unclear interpersonal struggle. At such times, the understanding
of states may be of great importance. In some therapies both parties
maintain a state in which no new undertakings are initiated, and in
which no progressive work is possible. Continual interpretations of
resistance may be useless or harmful unless they alter the state. It may
be helpful to determine the nature of this state and the warded-off states
that motivate its continued use. Examination of the role relationship
models and self-images that characterize this fruitless state may be useful
in reaching an understanding of how to modify controls so that a more
productive state can evolve.

UTILIZATION FOR THE WORKING MODELS OF THE PATIENT

Change occurs in increments and may repeat itself like an upward
spiral that swings back and forth across certain repeated vertical parallels. Patterns persist, yet they develop more adaptive forms. Each new
recognition of a pattern allows for greater choice; the pattern may be
modified, rather than entirely extinguished (Wheelis, 1973). Some aspects
of configurational analysis aid the therapist in communicating methods
for pattern recognition and helping the patient to attain a more pivotal
point for consciously altering habitual controls.

Ever since Joseph interpreted Pharaoh's dreams, patterns have been clarified so that they leap more starkly from communicated content. No radically novel technique is likely to be discovered after so much psychological history in the area of conversational interventions. But clearer, more incisive organization of information may develop, and some aspects of configurational analysis may permit more organized interventions of the kind that are already conventional.

STATE ANALYSIS

State analysis, as described in Chapter 2, is useful in clarifying existing patterns. While such clarification prepares the way for later interpretations explaining shifts in states, the state-labeling process is useful in its own right. The person gains distance from automatic repetitions of neurotic behavior when he is aware of the state he is in, was in, or is about to enter. When he recognizes a common sequence of transition between states, he can sometimes prevent movement into unproductive states. When he has already entered and is caught up in a disruptive state, and entangled in interlocking patterns of information, change is more difficult.

After sharing labels for states that are personally meaningful and evocative for the patient, rapid communication and attention to the larger significant patterns becomes necessary. This leads naturally into the next step of a sequence, the question of why a problem state comes about, and under what circumstances a desirable state becomes unstable and a shift occurs.

APPLICATION OF STATE IDENTIFICATION TO INTERVENTION DECISIONS IN CRISIS TREATMENT SETTINGS

One problem frequently encountered in a crisis clinic concerns the patient who is not in need of hospitalization but is in danger of committing acts that may seriously impair himself or others. The current crisis may be part of a turbulent series of events that occur not only because of their own intercausality but because of the personality characteristics of the individual. A brief period of psychotherapy may be indicated and facilities available, but the customary manner of working through conflicts or developmental impasses with neurotic patients is unlikely to be possible, at least at treatment onset. State analysis may provide a helpful paradigm for planning useful interventions.

The usual methods of psychodynamic psychotherapy are mainly effective when the person is in a working state and is capable of forming a therapeutic alliance (Langs, 1976). In the kind of situation described above, the person can be in alternative states. The goal of initial evaluation may be to work out not only the problem state but the likely state cycles. The patient is helped to avoid the most threatening states, and to gradually enter into a working state for increased periods of time. Other goals may lead to interventions that are premature.

For example, a young woman came to a special clinic for stress responses because of pressure from a friend who had stayed awake with her all night while she was in a state of suicidal depression. During the initial interview the patient was in a giddy state, characterized by *la belle indifference*, coquettish, inappropriate flirtatious behavior, and inability to maintain concentration on any topic. It was possible, however, to reconstruct events. Several weeks previously her mother had been killed in an automobile accident. She had managed to dispose of her mother's belongings, then turned for comfort to a boyfriend. After she had many periods of crying rage, he left her, saying that he had "not signed up for that sort of thing." She became suicidally depressed and took a sublethal dose of medication. She then called the second friend, who induced vomiting, spent the night with her, and finally was able to persuade her to come to the clinic. A potential state cycle involved *suicidal depression, crying rage, giddy and impulsive behavior*, and a *working* state. The *working* state in which the process might be cooperatively examined was not present at this time.

The initial paradigm of intervention was based on the goal of avoiding time in the *suicidal-depressed* state and increasing time in a potential *working* state. After even the preliminary evaluation, it was possible to understand that she was a dependent person who had never lived alone successfully. She was likely to enter impulsively into a liaison with a man, exchanging sex in the hope for comfort. When comfort was not forthcoming, as it was not likely to be in an impulsive liaison, she would enter a *crying rage*. The man would leave her. She would again enter a *suicidal depression*. It was also clear that if she returned to work in the *giddy* state she would probably be fired, as her situation was already tenuous.

The initial work was aimed at clarifying these state cycles and anticipating the initial steps that would lead to entry into them. The treatment agreement was constructed in the same manner. It was openly anticipated that the patient would find the therapist lacking in comfort, that she would impulsively miss hours. This possibility was described to her, and she was directed to return for a subsequent interview if it should happen. This plan included setting a limit on the number of therapy hours, having missed sessions count as one of those hours, and expecting that she would keep the next appointment, with no emotional penalty involved in having missed an hour.

During the course of therapy the time in the *depressed* state lessened and the suicidal intensity of that state decreased. *Giddy* and *impulsive* states occurred, the patient did set up impulsive liaisons, but was, in a way, partially anticipating the consequences and acting to reduce them. In therapy she developed a *working* state that occurred part of the time, spending other time in the *crying rage* state She was able to cooperate to some extent with the therapist, even in this latter state, since it was a predicted, prelabeled event and thus subject to discussion as part of the overall ground rules.

As control over states increased, and as the *working* state became more stable and frequent, it was possible to progress to the use of conventional clarifications and interpretations to help her make the next decisions in her life and to master recent events. During the *working* state in therapy she was able to establish a therapeutic alliance. She also learned that she had some control over her tendency to enter *suicidally depressed* and *impulsively giddy* states.

MODELS OF SELF-CONCEPTS AND ROLE RELATIONSHIPS

As just discussed for state analysis, selective use of self-concepts and role relationship models analyses may be useful for purposes of clarification and interpretation during the conduct of therapy. Such analyses were reviewed in Chapters 3 and 6, but Janice's therapy was not marked by the pointed use of these techniques. Of course, such interventions have been the cornerstones of psychodynamic interpretive technique and the clarifications of transactional analyses. Nonetheless, the use of models of multiple self-concepts and role relationship models, and the association of these schemata to particular states, may be an unusually clear manner of making such statements.

A common clinical instance where such techniques are useful occurs when the patient habitually presents a tale of multiple life events that have been experienced since the previous therapy interview, and is not doing so as an avoidance maneuver. The therapist may sense that there is a common thread of concern running through these reports but may have difficulty in locating it. The unifying theme may be found through recurrent models of role relationship and self-concepts. Similarly, patients sometimes talk repetitively about the traits and patterns they find in others. A useful focus on a target they can change is provided when the therapist helps them to see their own complementary roles and images.

Transference interpretations, especially those that provide a link between current reactions to the therapist and childhood role relationships with parents and siblings, are also sometimes clarified by a multiple role model approach. In order to obtain maximum change, it may be useful to simultaneously present the relationship model of the therapeutic alliance and that of the transference. As described earlier, this technique highlights the discrepancy between the transference model and other present and verifiable alternatives, and provides the patient with the optimal situation for change in inner belief systems through information processing.

Some patients have habitual difficulty in retaining such concepts. While the majority do well with verbal and nonverbal communications, some have a cognitive style that does not retain alternatives presented verbally long enough to permit decisive review and choice. In such instances, use of simple diagrams may facilitate a more visual form of information processing. Principally, role relationship models of self and other may sustain a concept for review over many situations. Such retention and referencing aids may be especially useful if role reversal is frequent, for that complexity confuses patients. With such aids a patient can see how the same model applies to the therapy situation, to current outside interpersonal relationships, to developmental experiences with past figures, and even to fantasy and dream relationships. This can also be carried forward in other forms such as art or movement therapy. Obviously, as with any technique such as free association or dream analysis, it can also prove to be divisive, or a waste of limited time.

INFORMATION PROCESSING

Finally, analysis of information processing patterns as discussed in Chapters 4 and 7 may lead to further clarifications. In the early days of psychoanalysis, interpretations were primarily directed toward uncovering unconscious wishes. Later, emphasis was placed on the importance to change of interpretation of defenses against unconscious wishes, so that the person might use conscious efforts to alter automatic and unconscious avoidances. **The configurational analysis approach goes beyond that, to suggest descriptions of the cognitive maneuvers by which the defensive operations are accomplished. Such descriptions** imply specific alternatives to current operations and give the patient an even better chance to alter controls by conscious choice.

For example, the patient may avoid the appropriate name for a sexual organ, using "it" instead. A general interpretation of defensive operations and warded-off contents might be "You avoid this topic because you are afraid that if we talk about sexual matters you will become excited." A more explicit statement of the cognitive maneuver plus a statement of the alternatives will center the patient more decisively at a point for conscious decision. Such an intervention might be worded as "You are afraid to say words like *penis, vagina,* and *vulva* because you are afraid that someone will become aroused if you do." This intervention says more explicitly what the patient is feeling, not doing. It says what the patient could do, in that the therapist is suggesting that the specific words be used and is modeling their use.

A brief vignette from a psychoanalysis reported elsewhere (Horowitz, 1977a) will illustrate this further.

When Mary was faced with a threatening situation she would control the progress of her thoughts by inhibiting representation of the threatening ideas and feelings. If this option failed, she would then inhibit translation of those ideas into other systems of representation (for example, she would not let image meanings translate into word meanings). She would also avoid associational connections. That is, she would use the first two maneuvers to avoid ideas and feelings that would be automatically elicited by information that had already gained representation. She would conclude a train of thought by early closure or by declaration of the impossibility of any solution. She would also change her attitude from active to passive, or vice versa, depending on the direction of greater threat.

Each of these maneuvers could be recognized as a conscious experience, although Mary did them unconsciously. Each operation could be explicitly interpreted in the context of some specific mental content and emotional response. With direction of attention to the flow of thought, she could become aware of what she was doing and try to do otherwise. A train of thought prematurely closed off could be resumed and further associations elaborated.

A complete working through of a unit of warded-off ideas and feelings would consist of several components. Usually, interpretation of each component was not necessary. The therapist simply said a few words to move matters along. These short phrases pointed out transference meanings, developmental linkages, relations to current events, avoidances, or warded-off ideas and feelings.

To illustrate the interpretation of cognitive maneuvers, an extended interpretive statement will be presented. The moment illustrated is derived from working through an erotic transference relationship. Mary had developed feelings of sexual excitement during the hour but was warding off recognition of such feelings. She was aware enough to communicate bodily sensations, but meanings of these self-perceptions went into and out of awareness. The interpretations were aimed at increased conscious status and acceptance of these and related meanings. A global interpretation is presented schematically in Table 22. In one column are phrases always spoken in isolation but grouped here in a series as if given as one long interpretation about a warded-off erotic transference response. In the second column is the function served by the phrase. The two cognitive interpretations were that she said, "I don't know," to prevent further representation of hazardous ideas, and that enactive representations of erotic excitement were not translated into words.

Table 22. Interpretative Phrases and Their Functions[a]

Phrase	Function
You say, "I don't know"	Specifies the behavior observed
So you won't go on thinking	Says what is accomplished by the behavior
You are feeling excited now	Labels the warded-off content
In your body	Calls attention to the mode of representation (bodily sensation) of the warded-off content and models its expression
You are afraid to know that in words	Identifies the cognitive maneuver of nontranslation; suggests translation
Because you think it is bad and dangerous	Calls attention to and labels motives for the warding off and suggests check to see if she does feel anxious or guilty
You felt the same way toward your father	Links the current ideas and feelings to a relevent role relationship model and its developmental basis
You felt it was bad and dangerous	Explains the original threat when warding-off maneuvers were desirable
The same thing happens with your male friends	Links the role relationship model underlying transference to current and past interpersonal patterns
Even though you do not consciously want to think of sexual excitement with them as bad and dangerous	Points out the incongruity between the old role relationship and her more ideal one

[a]From Horowitz (1977a, p. 371).

When Mary responded to such interpretive lines with introspective effort, she reexamined her immediate experience. Was she feeling excited or afraid? If she found such information—perhaps at the periphery of conscious representation—as images or bodily enactments, she tried to translate them into words, to allow associations, to stay with the topic. If she were alone, she would not behave this way. With the therapist she now felt safe enough and also pressured enough to counteract her automatic avoidances. The pressure came from the therapeutic alliance, since she rightly believed that she and the therapist shared a value placed on full representation and communication and from a transference role relationship model. She expected the therapist to be pleased and attentive if she cooperated with his wishes.

Whatever the weight of multiple motives, her conscious efforts to represent, to know, and to speak the previously unthinkable had a gradual effect. The warded-off complexes of ideas and feelings were found to be tolerable to her adult mind although they had been appraised as intolerable by her childhood mind. Avoidance was less necessary. She worked through warded-off complexes and also learned a new way of thinking by repeated trials of representation, and by cross-translation of image, enactive, and lexical representation.

Only partial changes in cognitive style occurred at any one time. Every major theme surfaced again and again, each time with additional nuances and greater clarity. During episodes of positive transference she could accept her erotic yearnings with complete understanding, as she could her anxieties and guilt feelings, her inclinations not to know, and the relevant associational networks.

CHOICE OF INTERVENTION TECHNIQUE

Once a specific control has been noted in relation to a problem where processing is avoided or distorted, the therapist may choose to intervene by interpretation or by direction of how processing should proceed. An interpretive intervention suggests a conceptual alternative that allows the patient to modify his controls if he so chooses. A directive **tells** the patient to modify his controls. The patient may take this as either a statement describing a useful procedure or as a kind of pressure that could threaten his independence. The therapist's choice between interpretation and suggestion must take into consideration the entire configuration, not only what will promote better information processing of a particular problem but also the relationship implications of that mutual endeavor.

The choice of how to tell a patient about a control that he can consciously shift is illustrated in Table 23. The hypothetical situation is one where a person is controlling the resolution of a potential flow of information by isolating meanings represented as visual images from word meanings. Sample control operations are listed in the left-hand column and examples of both interpretive and directive remarks are shown in separate columns in the appropriate rows. As noted above, the choice of interventions that are either **interpretive** or **directive** is a decision to be based on features of the patient's role sets, and the therapist's intuition of what is likely to aid progress and avoid transference expenses.

SUMMARY

While primarily a tool for the review and understanding of change processes after a period of therapy (or other intervention), configurational analysis can also be useful during therapy. After initial interviews, several of the early steps may assist the therapist in formulation and rational treatment planning. These procedures may be especially useful

Table 23. A Contrast between Interpretative and Directive Approaches to Changing Controls[a]

Control	Interpretation	Direction
Inhibiting translation of images into words	"You do not let yourself describe the images you are having because you are afraid to think clearly about them and talk about them."	"Describe your images to me in words." "Tell me what that image means."
Inhibiting translation of words into images	"You do not let yourself see that idea visually because you are afraid of the feelings that might occur if you did."	"Form a visual image about that idea and report it to me."
Inhibiting intensification of vague images	"You are afraid to let that fleeting image become really clear in your mind because you are afraid you will feel bad if you do."	"Try to hold onto those images and sharpen them."

[a]From Horowitz (1978, p. 340).

during ongoing therapy as a means for exploring the causes and solutions to periods of impasse. Some aspects of state analysis, modeling of self-images and relationships, and understanding information-processing styles may be directly useful with the patient as clarifications and interpretations of patterns that can be changed.

Transcript Illustrations

A. RELATIONSHIP PROCESSES: THE THERAPEUTIC ALLIANCE

Establishment of a therapeutic alliance was a marked feature of the therapy with Janice because of difficulties imposed by her style of pretending, the interaction of her style with the special clinical situation, and the resulting vagueness of focus for the therapeutic communication. The alliance was developed gradually, reaching its peak by the eighth hour of therapy, as described in Chapter 6. Excerpts from transcripts illustrate the process of developing this alliance and counteracting tendencies to establish either a social relationship or the types of positive and negative transferences discussed in Chapter 6. In what follows, more "raw data" are presented to allow the reader to form his or her own opinions, and the author discusses the line of reasoning behind his interventions after each segment of dialogue. The order is sequential, from the first to the last of the 12 hours of therapy.

PRETENSE

A style of pretense leading to the *tra-la-la* state has been described. It prevented Janice from using the therapy to master her current life problems. Instead of experiencing herself as the subject of a thought and feeling as she did when her self-concept was that of a learner, she experienced herself, when pretending confidence, as part of the audience at her own performance. This stance was familiar to her and she described it in the first evaluation interview. She said, "I can go for help, I can go through the motions, I can impress people with my intelligence and my ability and my, I don't mean, togetherness, ah, self-recognition or whatever."

The evaluator picked this up, "So you were afraid that somehow, even here, you could fool the therapist."

And the patient said, "Yes." She continued, "It's like when you're a kid, and you're crying because you're sad, and all of a sudden you get involved with how the tears are going down your cheek or something."

THE PROBLEM OF AN AGREED-UPON FOCUS OF CONCERN

The initial attempt to establish a focus occurred after about 10 minutes of the first hour of therapy. Janice had been talking about the unreality of her brother's death and how she felt she was warding off feelings of sadness. The therapist clarified by suggesting that she wanted the therapy to make the event seem so real to her that she could then experience grief. Note that she did not agree with his attempt to clarify, and tried to expand the focus for the therapeutic effort.

P: Well, you know, it's not just like [pause] part of it is—is that I don't believe it's true, it isn't real and I'm working very hard to make it stay unreal.
T: Uhhuh. And if our work were to make it real it would be painful for you.
P: MmHumm. MmHum.
T: But you think we should do that.
P: I'm not sure I do.
T: MmHmm.
P: I'm not, I mean I'm here.
T: But now that you're here it's a little like being in the hot seat . . .
P: [Laughs].
T: And you'd like to get out of it?
P: Well, I'm going to go through with it, I mean you know I've had a couple chances to back out and the fact that I haven't says to me that this is something that's important. If's not just Sam [her dead brother], it's, you know, it goes back. I've been depressed, and depressed about being depressed for a long time and it's time to do something about it.
T: Well, in a way, working on the reality, as painful as it is, of Sam, might be just a first step for you to see what the process is like.
P: MmHm.
T: And you can decide if you wanted to go any further.
P: I like that word "reality," cause that's what I want. I want to be able to accept and see and feel reality and I, I've been living in a very unreal world [pause]. And you know, like I say, it makes everything kind of fuzzy, kind of foggy, softens the edges a little bit [pause]. And um, it makes my perceptions unreal and [pause] it, it's confusing, it's hard to maintain, too. It takes a lot of energy. I'm tired all the time [pause] and [pause] just, I can't be creative. I, I've been talking about being a composer all my life, and I

finally got some time, and an opportunity to do it, and it, I, I, I don't even write down little tunes anymore.

In the above excerpt from transcripts, the therapist did not catch the meaning of her reluctance to focus on the stressful event, when, in response to his question about wanting to work together to make it real she said, "I'm not sure I do." In his statement, "But now that you're here it's a little like being in the hot seat," he was going along with the idea that she was warding off grief because she feared the intensity of her feelings. He did not recognize her concern with seeking therapy for reasons that were not related to the death of her brother.

The patient attempted to show him what she believed was the right track when she said, "It's not just Sam, it's, you know, it goes back. I've been depressed, and depressed about being depressed for a long time." The therapist, however, perhaps already worried by a diffusion in focus, and concerned with participating in a televised teaching–research document as well as a therapy, persisted in trying to establish the contract around the stress event. In retrospect, this persistent effort to set a focus was viewed by the patient as his inability to see beyond her pretenses, and by the therapist as an error in timing. He did allow some space for other matters when he said, "As painful as it is [working on the death], it might be just a first step for you to see what the process [of psychotherapy] is like."

As it happened, this was just about where the patient wanted to be. It was why she responded positively, saying she liked the word "reality" and "that's what I want." The therapist had not insisted that they drop the topic of her brother's death, her "ticket of admission" to the stress clinic, and focus on other problems in her life; nor had he indicated that he was going to devote himself exclusively to the stress event. She hoped a working relationship was possible and so continued to give more information about herself. She said that she was living in an unreal world, that she was confused, tired all the time, and not creative or self-activated, but she did not provide a clear sense of her goals for therapy.

That is why, about 10 minutes later, the therapist again tried to see if they could agree on a focus.

T: Now, how would it be if we were to just focus our mission on the issue of learning the meaning of the news that your brother had died?
P: Accepting it and saying it's real?
T: Yeah.

P: And, and you think that that would um [pause] kind of open up [pause], like, the way you said it would make me, teach me how to do it for the rest of the stuff?

T: No, I don't think it would do everything for you. I think if you, if you wanted to explore your style of living, where you are in your life course, that might be a matter that would take much longer. But it might be dealing with the first thing that's happened to you that's brought you into therapy.

P: Mm.

T: And it might give you more information about yourself, what therapy is like. And then you could decide if you wanted anything else.

P: I want an instant solution [laughs].

T: MmHm.

P: I want [pause].

T: Well, I wish I could give you one [an instant solution].

P: Yeah, I know. I tried helping the relatives of the old people I work with and I had to stop 'cause my godmother complex overwhelmed me; I always wanted to wave my wand and have everybody be all right [long pause]. Um, I don't want to. I don't want to, the, I mean, the other stuff is a little more detached. I'm more used to it, it's been going on for a long time. But I don't want to say, "Yes, let's go ahead and convince me that Sam is really dead." Um, the fact that I don't want to so much says to me that I probably should [focus on Sam's death].

T: Well, I wouldn't go ahead with that [focus on Sam's death] unless you agreed to it [long pause]. Well, we can leave that an open issue, come back to it.

P: Oh, it sounded kind of like an ultimatum.

T: No.

P: No? [long pause] Well I, I do really want to [long pause]. It's an intellectually wanting to.

T: MmHm.

P: Just [pause] I, I um, don't want to keep putting all the energy into avoiding it.

Note how carefully in the above segment both patient and therapist circle around the issue of having an agreed-upon aim; it is a quite subtle interaction. The therapist asked how it would be if the focus was just on the meaning to her of the death. She didn't say yes or no. Instead, she asked a question. She hoped to elicit more information about the therapist and avoid having to answer his question. The therapist gave a brief answer to hold her to the topic. She went on asking the therapist, "and you think that would kind of open up, teach me to do it for the rest of the stuff"? That is, she was trying to get the therapist to promise her a more extensive therapy goal, a test for a possible entry of the therapist as a rescuer, one of the positive transference potentials described in Chapter 6. The therapist caught on and disagreed; he could not offer everything.

She then went on to obscure the matter. It was clear enough when she said, "But I don't want to say, 'Yes, let's go ahead and convince me that Sam is really dead.' " That line should have continued with her saying what at the moment was closer to her authentic inner experience. "What I really want to do is talk to you about why I can't go on to develop myself, my work, my love life." Instead she undid her refusal to focus on the death by saying, "I don't want to talk about Sam but I probably should because I don't want to," implying that her reluctance was probably only a defense against the intensity of her feelings about it. While she was not aware of it, this was also a repetition need to relive the funeral and have it come out differently. **This** time she would cry and not be silly or withdrawn. With reenactment, however, the same dangers could return: She would not be sad, and would be in danger of pretending or withdrawing.

The therapist noted her undoing maneuvers. He countered them by saying, "I wouldn't go ahead with that unless you agreed to it." There was then a long pause in which glances were exchanged. This pause and the glances tested the therapist's solidity in demanding her agreement to any focus. The therapist ended this contest of wills by saying, "Well, we can leave that an open issue."

By her response, "It sounded like an ultimatum," the patient indicated that she had experienced the episode as a contest of wills. By saying it was not an ultimatum, the therapist indicated that he was firm but did not demand submission. He indicated his real position, his willingness to go on exploring the issue with her. She then said she wanted to agree to a focus on the death of Sam. But this too was inaccurate. She undid the statement again by saying, "It's only an intellectual wanting to." Her agreement about the focus on Sam was probably an effort to conciliate, that is, to move from a *competitive* state toward a more mutual *working* state. But the movement is incomplete; pretense remains.

Even with lack of agreement on a therapeutic focus there was a chance for her to test the therapist. She realized that he was not going to let her avoid the issues by agreeing to a very diffuse contract in which he would, in effect, promise her too much. By avoiding either pitfall he became a safer, real, and more reliable figure.

SECOND THERAPY HOUR

At the onset of the second hour, she indicated the presence of a misalliance around the theme of being treated for a stress-response syndrome. That she reported the misalliance indicated her wish to receive authentic treatment and her growing partial trust in the therapist. It was a further challenge to the therapist to see if he could form a therapeutic alliance or if he would fulfill her transference wishes and fears.

P: Um. You know what ha-happened when I walked downstairs last week thinking [pause] he wants me to cry, you know?
T: I want you to cry?
P: You want me to cry, that you would be successful in a, you know the therapy would be successful when I cried, when I broke down and said, "Yes, my brother's dead," and cried about it you know? Like, like uh, what's his stake in it? You know, he's gotta, he's gotta, he's the big man, and it's very important and it's for the students [a reference to being televised] and, I have to perform.
T: Now it sounds like I have to perform.

The therapist did not reject the role she outlined for him. This permitted her to go into it further.

P: Yeah! Right! Right you, have to succeed by being incredible, and by curing me in, in, curing me, right [laughs], in four, three or, something sessions and I have to perform by breaking down and crying.
T: Yeah. But it would be kind of like **my** success and **you'd** be kind of like a puppet?
P: MmHm, MmHm. And, and you know, I mean there's a lot in me that would do that, that would, that **would** perform. And, and, you know, ah, specially if it would, like, get you off my back, get **me** off my back for a while, you know. So that I could **do it all on the surface** and ah [pause] or something like that [pause]. So I, I wanted to say that, but I wanted to, ah, talk to you about it and get some kind of feel for you.
T: Right.

Note that the patient recognized her alienation from her experience as she said, "I could do it all on the surface." She is telling the therapist how she will only pretend to work in therapy; she is asking him to counter this and make therapy real for her despite her style, her resistances, and the artifacts introduced by televising and having a potential audience. This is her effort toward forming the therapeutic alliance.

P: So that I wouldn't feel that way about you. Uh, but I didn't, I didn't go beyond saying, you know, beyond that. Like, I didn't have any specific questions to ask.
T: But that would be important to do because unless we have a feeling that we're working as a team in some way that's useful to you.
P: [Interrupts] Right.

T: Then you'd go with this idea that I was going to do a peformance for students.

The therapist is not saying anything here that she does not know but in saying it he (1) indicates that these matters should be discussed, (2) shows he understands her dilemma and includes her positive wish for a useful experience, and (3) sets up a contrast between the possible therapeutic alliance and her fears about setting up other relationships in which she would be compliant and used. While the therapist did not know it yet, she feared complying with her mother, submitting to her values, and hence rebelled at the funeral. Were the therapist authoritarian he would have repeated patterns she experienced with her parents. Transference is often pinned to realities, and patients provoke such realities in their therapy.

She goes on in the *tra-la-la* state to set up a fantasy where she and the therapist can take that which she fears as humor.

P: [Shouting] And you know like I could see it! I could just see it! Here's, and she finally she breaks down and she cries, and between her fingers she sees the doctor kind of go . . . [she nods with a superior look].
T: I win.
P: Yeah, so it seems. So um, w—I figured I'd better say something about it right away or it would be useless coming at all [pause, sigh]. My other, um fear that I have about this particular situation is ah [pause] that because you're a man you won't really understand me. You know, that sexism will get in your way. That, um [pause] that you will try to elicit the responses that a feminine woman is supposed to have or something like that.

Because the therapist has been reasonably perceptive and reliable, she is able to state further fears of him, especially since she already believes they are not valid. She is checking further to see if he can stand challenging statements without retaliating by one-upping her or becoming anxious over lack of competence to be helpful. That is, this test serves as a check to see if the therapist can be unlike her mother, neither telling her how to be a woman nor crushed by her disagreement with him.

Later in the second session there is another example of the process of establishing the alliance. She had been talking in generalities that continued to relate to a social rather than therapeutic relationship. The therapist then referred to her fears that he, a male therapist, would inflict his definition of female identity upon her. As known from the material that emerged later in therapy, and as just noted above, this theme was important to one of her role relationships. She was still engaged in a developmental struggle to separate from her mother, she wanted to avoid returning home to her, to avoid identification with her, and also to avoid hurting her mother as she left childhood to become her own person. She was not really afraid of male chauvinism in the therapist; she thought he might be all right and was testing to see if he was. The therapist sensed that such concerns rode upon the realistic issues of the usefulness of clinicians of the opposite sex for patients and he demonstrated a willingness to examine openly, and in dialogue, her concerns about him.

T: Yeah. So your concerns are realistic, too, I mean, this **is** being recorded, male psychiatrists **have** been accused of making various projections onto women, those things are all true.

P: Mmm. Yeah. I don't, um [pause] really feel **that** um [pause] um, you know. In fact I mind **that** more than I mind the fact that it's being recorded.

T: MmHm. I don't quite get what you mean. [She meant she did not mind being recorded, she minded his being male. He did not follow this.]

P: I mind the fact that you're a male psychiatrist.

T: MmHm.

P: You know like I, I don't think it applies to all men [pause] maybe it does a little bit. You know, that I don't expect men to really be able to understand or I expect them to leap to the wrong conclusion and . . .

T: MmHm.

P: Like you said, to project.

T: So, one thing you're worried about is that you'll be maybe hyperalert to what I'm doing and won't be able to—

P: [interrupts] I'm doing this on so many levels, I mean it.

T: MmHm.

P: That's exactly right. I mean I'm sitting here and I'm watching you and I'm recording what you're doing. [She may be more sensitive to recording than she knows and says, and here turns the tables: a role reversal; she records and can later judge him.]

T: MmHm.

P: And I'm judging it, you know on a couple different levels as far as your relationship to me and what I think you'd like and whether or not I like you and whether or not, you know, you're a good, good shrink. And then I'm watching what I say and hearing it, you know, is this new, did I know that, how I feel about this, how that looks.

T: And that's probably one of your characteristic traits, isn't it?

P: That I do things on different levels?

T: Yuh.

P: Yeah, that's why it's so exhausting for me.

T: Right.

This was an "agreement point"; they agreed that she did things on many levels, meaning that the surface communication and her authentic inner experience were disjunctive. She was reassured that the therapist could know this, she became excited about the possibility of a therapeutic alliance when she revealed, "I'm doing this on so many levels."

P: I do, it's, I [voice loud] don't like parties or groups because it's just too much, and I, and I'm watching all the um, it's okay if I can just watch. It, it's interesting in fact to watch the dynamics between people and what's going on at a surface level and what's going on underneath and [trails off].
T: Mm.
P: When I have to be part of it sometimes it's a very painful.
T: Hard for you to get your heart into things then.
P: I've been turning it off.

She went on to talk about some troublesome interactions with Phillip. Something about this sounded authentic although her communication abounded in generalizations. The therapist picked out a theme and attempted to focus on her fear of leaving a relationship she saw as excessively dependent because she would then feel too alone.

T: Yuh. But at the center of the story you'll be alone.
P: MmHm. Mm. That's interesting [very long pause]. I do feel really alone. [pause]. I'm constantly reassuring myself that everybody loves me, I mean listing, ticking off . . .
T: Hm.
P: I don't know, like they [voice almost a whisper].

At this point she oscillated between a *hurt and not working* and *hurt but working* state. As a resistance to going deeper into a painful topic she went on to speak in generalities.

P: It's like, I'm sitting here saying [voice normal], "I know they do" [love her]. I know it, if this is something I know, I don't have to question it. And if I have them, then I don't need, uh, you know. Like I really need to go out and have lots of friends [pause], which is my explanation of why I haven't been, um [pause] trying to get close friends out here [pause].

She did not trust the therapist enough to tell him how friendless she felt at this point because she feared both her own defective self-image and having him see her as defective. She went on to describe other matters of current concern. The therapist noted this but said nothing about it. As she resumed a clearer line of speech, she began to talk about feeling that her work degraded her. The therapist then responded and tried to clarify her expectations that he too would regard her as a defective or bad, that if she let go of her avoidances she would expose herself to self-disgust. She contemplated this briefly, then stayed with it but entered the *tra-la-la* state to avoid emotional confrontation with the ideas.

T: So, with this kind of idea you're vulnerable to feeling kind of degraded.
P: MmHm [long pause].
T: Well, how about, how about being a patient here? Does that have any connotation of being degraded?
P: MmHm [pause]. It does and it doesn't. I mean I've been a lot happier since, since making the decision of actually coming here.
T: MmHm.
P: And, and, like all this past week I went around feeling happy and feeling good, and you know a little stronger and stuff. And I knew that it was because I had done something that I hope will be good for me. But at the same time I, yeah, I don't go around telling everybody. Like I'm not going to tell my family. To them that would be degrading [enters *tra-la-la* state]. "What's wrong with you? You don't talk to outsiders. You don't. Oh you're so weird, you're always so weird" [pause]. And uh, I make a joke out of it when I tell my friends. "Guess what! Tra-la-la-la and for free! Tra-la-la-la tra-la and I'm on tape!" That aspect of it, you know, nothing about why and [trails off].
T: Yeah, well, that sounds a little like you're telling them not to take it seriously.
P: MmHm.
T: It's just a lark.
P: MmHm, MmHm. I'm not allowed to take it seriously.
T: Yuh.
P: Why am I here? In fact I almost didn't come today. I'm, I don't need to go here.

She had an improved but temporary image of the therapist and so trusted him not to criticize her when she revealed new information about almost not coming for the session. The therapist did not criticize her. He interpreted the meaning.

T: Yuh. Well, you're afraid to take it [the opportunity for therapy] seriously.
P: Yuh. And, and, all I can say, you know, like I can't say "There's something wrong with me." I can't, well for one thing, that's, that, you know, that's the . . . always too dramatic, right? If I sat down and I said, "I'm really worried and I'm really unhappy," and uh part of me would say [whispers], "Oh, wow, there she goes again. She loves being center stage."

T: Uh huh.

P: And so I have to say, well, it's 'cause I'm tired of being depressed and I know there's some things I want to change and I know I can't do it myself. So this is one way of doing it. And that's what I say. And that's what I say, if anything, to my friends. I think that's what I said to Phillip. You know he was really concerned. I just kind of popped in and said, "Oh, guess what I'm going to start doing." And he said, "Oh," and he kind of came back a few minutes later and he was really concerned, "Why are you doing this?"

T: Mm.

P: "I didn't know you were unhappy," he didn't say that but, you know.

T: Yuh. **He** took it seriously.

P: MmHm. And so I told him, "Well, you know, I've been depressed. You remember this, you remember that and I can't do it by myself so I'm going to do it." And he accepted that [pause]. And, and, I mean I wasn't going to tell him [pause] anything else [pause]. See I'm not even going to say it now [laugh, pause].

T: Well, I'm not going to force you to either.

By interpreting her fears the therapist indicated he would not be wishy-washy or fooled. He also indicated that he would not be dictatorial or authoritarian. He set boundaries appropriate to a therapeutic alliance.

P: Yeah. Well see I still feel like I'm, I'm being dramatic. "What is she keeping under cover? What can't she even admit to herself? [Dramatically said] Tune in next week!"

T: That might be right.

P: [Laughs]. That just goes with the feeling of unreality, I can't even evaluate myself.

T: Yeah. Well, look, you've been checking up on both of us and this situation and it's a style of yours. You know that a style of yours is to be very private and secret, I think.

P: You know, one of the tools I use to do that, is to act very, very open.

T: Mm.

P: I'm more open than anybody I know as far as what I'll say about myself and, and . . .

T: Yuh, yuh.

P: And I go around embarrassing people 'cause I tell their secrets, too.

T: Yuh.

P: [Histrionically] And, "Oh I didn't know you wanted that kept private." But it's a cover-up.

T: Yuh.

P: I've known that. I've just never said it.

T: Yuh, well you're keeping things from yourself, too.

P: MmHm.

T: So it's natural that you start out by checking out the situation, testing me,
     testing yourself, and what's going on and . . .

P: Mm.

T: That's okay. Why not? We'll see if we can work together. It's a trial, really.
     I think that's realistic.

P: I'm glad you said that, 'cause I've been aware of that with people like,
     especially in a relationship like a boyfriend or also now, like how far can
     they go? How much can this person take?

T: Yuh.

P: Can he take me being, really being mean? [long pause]

T: Okay, well, we are going to have to stop now, and go on next week at the
     same time.

THIRD THERAPY HOUR

Arriving at a level where there is discussion of her inner experiences
rather than her customary presentations to others is an important part
of establishing a therapeutic alliance with this patient and is further
illustrated in session three. At one point she offered a kind of intellec-
tualized self-interpretive statement that she was trying to fail at work
in order to hurt her parents. While this might have been accurate, she
was not experiencing her life that way. The therapist had been focusing
on what she experienced rather than her intellectual interpretations of
what might be going on. He pointed out that she was not experiencing
ideas of revenge against her parents. This may have been an error. Janice
did feel she was hurting her mother by pursuing independence in her
own way. If the therapist had recognized this at the time, he might have
clarified that location of the meaning of "hurting her parents" and corrected the distortion of meaning that led, in part, to the inauthentic
quality of her expressions at this time.

In this test, the therapist attempted to focus on her immediate
experiences about work. The sequence was first a feeling that she didn't
have to get to work on time, and could let herself arrive late. That led
to reprimands and risked loss of her employment. Then she became
self-critical and wondered what was happening to her. The patient argued
that when the time came to get ready to go to work, she had the feeling
that it would come out okay, and this somehow contributed to a foggy
feeling.

The therapist said, "And the foggy feeling is like nothing really
counts." The patient agreed. The therapist then related this pattern to
the treatment by saying: "You're worried about coming to see me. Isn't
it right, too, that you'll treat **this** as though it doesn't really count?" She
confirmed the pattern as she responded, "You know, it's funny, **I have**

to do that and every time I admit to myself that it **does** count very much, I start to do all these things to prove that its not true."

She went on to talk about her feeling that she was not allowed to **really** be in therapy, that she was dramatizing herself by coming for it. This statement led directly to the statement that she had come for therapy because she could not get hold of her life, that she had used the death of her brother as a ticket of admission. After the therapist said that, the session went on in the following way. She became excited because she anticipated that the misalliance of "false pretenses" could be resolved, without criticism or dissolution of the therapy. In terms of relationship models, she was excited because she envisioned a possibility that the therapist could be a safe teacher who would understand both her wish to learn and her fear of exposing her need to learn.

P: [Excited] Yeah, see, that's the thing. I constantly feel guilty that you guys are making more of that than I am—
T: Uh-huh.
P: And I . . .
T: You wanted to come to therapy **anyway**.
P: I wanted to come to therapy anyway, I did. And if that'll get me in, fine. And I, and I keep saying you know, but . . .
T: Then you feel it's false pretenses.
P: Yeah, I do, and I say, well, I, or I won't say anything about it because maybe it is, you know . . .
T: Um.
P: I mean, it did happen, it really did happen and I **really don't feel a thing about it** and that really bothers me.
T: Yeah. But it also was enough. It was just enough [pressure on you] that you could then get yourself to therapy.
P: But see I can't accept that.
T: Well, then when you start thinking seriously that you really want therapy, for a moment that frightens you. And then you have to run all over the place.
P: Uh-huh [long pause, sniff, pause]. I am a hypochondriac in that I really try to get **out** of things, so many times it's easier **not** to do anything, and uh [pause] I always want to stay home from work or school or whatever.
T: Un-huh.

A few minutes later the clarification of "false pretenses" continued.

T: Yeah, but you see, you have various predictions about this. One prediction is that I am going to somehow follow you into your brother's death. . . .
P: Uh-huh.

T: And that'll miss the point because that's not what's causing your suffering right now.
P: That's right.
T: So that would just be a waste of time.
P: Uh-huh.
T: And you'll have lost one of your only opportunities.
P: That's right. How did you know that? I mean that, you know, this whole question. I guess I expect you not to know that.
T: Well, you've been telling me, else I wouldn't know.

This is accurate and an attempt by the therapist to use clarity to substantiate the growing therapeutic alliance. Because the patient paused for a long time, the therapist continued his statement.

P: [Long pause].
T: See, your other theory is that you won't tell me these things.
P: I'm surprised that you said I've been telling you.
T: Yeah, trying to.
P: [Long pause] I'm so used to people seeing my surface words that sound so deep and really aren't.
T: Yeah, but you've also been telling me to watch out. You've been waving red flags and saying watch out, don't take the surface, please don't.
P: Yeah. Yeah.
T: You're communicating.
P: Oh good [long pause]. Please don't be impressed by my surface [long pause]. It's funny to ask people to do that when you're throwing out a surface that says so clearly that you're impressed [pause].
T: Well, there's a great danger for you in working. Somewhere, I don't know exactly what the words are, but it's that I would somehow be disgusted by you [long pause].
P: Hm. [Pause]. I don't think I thought about [pause] that, other than in symbolic terms, you as a symbol of anybody who sees beneath the surface.
T: Yeah.
P: You in your capacity as uh doctor sitting here in this chair, not knowing me in my outside life, I have the most fear of that, I think, than otherwise. [pause]. I expect *you* to be able to take more.
T: Yeah, well, you have a right to have that expectation.
P: [Sighing].
T: I mean it's true.
P: Isn't it funny—Isn't it funny, everything's—People think they're so disgusting and they're neat [sniff].

She went on to be more open about her impairments, referring to her laziness and criticizing herself for lack of direction. As the hour closed, the therapist again attempted to arrive at an agreed-upon therapeutic focus.

P: [Coughing, sniff] Or—or like saying, well, so I'm lazy. So what? So what's so bad about being lazy? You know? I mean, obviously I think there is something really really **bad** about being lazy. But I'm trying to be accepting. I'm trying to say, "Okay, I'll let myself be lazy at times."

T: Oh **there** is something you **do** experience. You experience yourself as being lazy sometimes.

P: Uh-huh.

T: It gets you into trouble and it **does** scare you.

P: Uh-huh. You mean that's a real feeling that I really know I really have?

T: We could really find out something about that because it's a real feeling that you really have and there's real events and you can trace them.

P: Hm. I try to—to say, now, this is not laziness, this is a need or I'm mad and I'm dealing with a problem or something like that, but it all goes under the heading of laziness, and in some instances is more excusable than in others. These are times when staying in bed and reading a book is okay. I'm coping or something like that, or recharging, or whatever. And there are times when it's just plain not okay or if I've done enough coping.

For a time the therapist took on the responsibility for arriving at and maintaining a focus. He tentatively defined this to Janice as dealing with bad self-images around her current developmental crises of living independently. Here is an example for that kind of effort, one in which he used mild sarcasm to undercut her generalities and make the point that the therapy was to be about **her.**

P: If people like each other, everything else would work out [sigh]. If people act the way they're supposed to act, then—then the rest of the world should just fall into place [pause]. If Gloria treats me [pause] in an understanding and open and [pause] everything-fine way, then it should continue that way [pause]. Well, it certainly can't be **my** fault.

T: Of course not.

P: But it changed.

T: Of course it did. No, in psychotherapy we **never** look for the things that the person has about themselves that they could change because . . .

P: [Laughing].

T: That hurts people's feelings.

P: They have to change—circumstances.

T: Changing the **outside** world is what **we** focus on.

P: Yeah, let's have a revolution. Make me a king [pause]. That's an interesting choice of words, isn't it? [Long pause] I certainly would rather be king than queen.

T: Right.
P: [Long pause] I don't have all the status I want [pause].
T: Well, it's very painful to be humiliated, and I think you're experiencing many things in your everyday life maybe as a humiliation. Whatever twenty-five means to you, it's a milestone. Symbolically and at different times earlier in your life, you had fantasies about the future, and expectations of what you'd be doing about now.
P: Yes.

FIFTH THERAPY HOUR

That type of interchange was repeated many times before a therapeutic relationship became firmly established. Another example is found in the fifth therapy hour. Once again the therapist tried to define the therapeutic alliance. This consisted of saying the obvious, and also repeating what had already been said in order to help the patient maintain it clearly in mind, as a contrast to other relationship possibilities. In the following excerpt, the therapist said that his role was to listen, to try to help as best he could, and to understand the meanings of what she was saying. Note that this was followed by a long pause, followed by the patient challenging what the therapist had said. She asked for more, in effect. With another type of patient the therapist might interpret or remain silent to create working anxiety. With this patient the therapist felt it important to let her hear him repeat the refrain.

P: Huh [pause] okay [sigh, long pause]. I wonder, I don't know why I always, I feel this compulsion [pause] to talk. I, I was, I think I told you, I'm not sure, I was in a T group class once in college. And—uh—[pause] we were supposed to be studying theory but it was mainly, we went to class and there was a T group, and I always had to talk, had to start the thing, had to be responsible. I wasn't the leader or anything, but if everybody sat there and didn't say anything [pause] I had to bring up something.
T: Well, that's no secret. Here that's your responsibility.
P: [Pause] Why do I feel so funny about it? Maybe I feel it **is** a secret [long pause] [enters competitive state]. It's all up to me, huh? [pause] If I talk or I don't talk, or [pause]. What would you do if I didn't talk?
T: I'd ask you why you weren't talking.
P: Mm.
T: I mean, that is, our rules are that you'll talk.
P: Uh-huh.

T: My role is that I'll listen and try and help you as best I can to understand the meanings of what you're saying and not saying [long pause].

P: When does helping me to understand what I'm saying and feeling turn into helping me to change? Does it happen automatically or do I start trying to do something? [pause]

T: Well, if you understand things more clearly, it puts you in kind of a pivotal position where you can change. There are some occasions where therapists give advice, but that's not what **we're** going to do. That is, I'm basically going to try to just understand what's going on and help **you** understand what's going on, and leave the decisions about **what** to change up to you. But you know we're—uh—we're in a position now where you came in and your first complaint was that you weren't reacting to the fact that your brother died. And then it turns out that you were interested in therapy for some time, but also very reluctant. . . .

P: Uh-huh.

T: . . . to come in and in a way the way **you** were experiencing it, you were using that as an excuse. . . .

P: Uh-huh.

T: . . . to come in, I **guess** because you were afraid that, uh, it would be humiliating to come in just because you wanted help . . .

P: Well—

T: . . . with that.

P: I feel that, it's not really legitimate. I don't really feel badly enough. Well, I **constantly** feel that way. I'm not sick enough to stay home, you know, when I feel bad. So, you ask me how I feel. I complain about menstrual cramps or something. "How do you feel?" [and dramatically, louder] "well, I don't feel **terrible**" [voice back to normal].

This led, again, to a discussion of the therapeutic contract and a focus on bad self-concepts, especially as they centered around episodes connected with the death of her brother. She repeated that she had been conscious of using the death of her brother as an excuse for coming to get therapy and also as a way of getting sympathy from other people. The therapist said that telling other people had been experienced by her as faking it, as cheating people out of their sympathy. She then went back and forth as to whether or not she had been upset about her brother's death. Then the therapist interpreted this defense by saying: "You take one position and then you take another position and you don't know which position you're taking to get the **other** person to take a position and which position is **your** position." This type of intervention generally caused her to shift from the *tra-la-la* to a *hurt but working* state.

It is indicative of a partial therapeutic alliance that the patient was able to laugh and say "Yes" to this. The therapist continued:

T: And you don't know when you're manipulating somebody or when you're presenting yourself honestly. You feel both ways.

P: Exactly. And I can turn around and argue both sides of the case with, with [pause] you know, like a deep-down feeling or something. This is the truth, I was for real. Or, or, like that. I'm manipulating you or I'm not manipulating you. I can, it, it often depends on the mood I'm in at the time, how I see my behavior [pause]. And I have to fight a lot and I have to see it as disgusting.

T: Yeah.

P: And, well, if I was in a bad mood, I could say [louder] tra-la-la-la. And say it and then, and then, and then shelve it.

Establishing a therapeutic alliance is not just something that has to be done so that therapy work can **then** be done. For many patients, as for Janice, it is the work of therapy, or one aspect of it, to set up this relationship because it requires developmental progress to trust another, allow intimate communication, and accept feedback without disgrace.

Later in this, the fifth hour, she spoke of the importance to her of the therapist not falling for things that she said.

P: I'm really glad you haven't fallen for a lot of the stuff I've said, and you know, images I've thrown at you because [pause] the minute you fell for those and started treating me like I was really together or really intelligent and really any of the other things that so many people think, I would lose respect for you.

T: Um.

P: Because uh [long pause].

T: There are two ways for us to walk **off** a useful path for you. One would be for me to think of you as the "cat's meow." And the other would be for me to be critical of you in any way. I'll try not to do either of those things.

P: That's nice. Really—I mean, I sit here and I say, "Well, you just sit there and nod," but at the same time it's good because you sit there and nod and you say something that makes me think about . . .

T: Um.

P: . . . what I've just said or whatever [long pause] that, that's uh [pause] that's fine with me [long pause].

T: Okay. That's fine with me.

This is another "point of agreement" that builds a base from which risks can be taken. Nonetheless, it was difficult for her to give up her avoidance maneuvers.

SEVENTH THERAPY HOUR

In the seventh interview the therapist confronted her with her diffusion of their focus by bringing up the issue of termination at the end of the following month, timed to give them five additional sessions. He then continued to confront her with the diffusion of focus and its function as a defense. Later, he interpreted a focus on bad images of herself as related to her brother's death. He related the laziness in herself about which she felt disgust to her behavior in the therapy as she attempted to postpone tackling central issues.

T: Well, you see we're just hovering at a level of abstraction with, where there's no specifics. I understand what you mean, and I sympathize with you. You do want to change. But your mind turns away from the issue of what it is you would like to change.

P: Well, you picked one that keeps popping into my mind now. You said that you weren't going to talk about it—laziness. [This is, incidentally, an example of her use of externalization: the therapist is the one who won't talk of her disapproved traits.] This is what I keep thinking of when I think of specific behavior I'd like to change. I'd like to not want to lie around so much. I'd like to not need to read so much. I'd like to not sleep so much and eat so much and, and [pause] be capable of doing so much nothing.

T: Um. But you see—well, I'm going to exaggerate what you just said in a way. I'll exaggerate to this: You were saying to me right now, "Make me not want to be lazy."

P: Um-hm.

T: "Not want to read so much. Make me not want to . . ." I can't make you not want to.

P: Um-hm. But, see, following what I was saying about the change coming inside first and then outside, if I feel that if I had a more acceptable image of myself that I just naturally wouldn't want to. 'Cause all that is just to get away from . . .

T: More acceptable than what?

P: In what, do you mean?

T: More acceptable **than** what?

P: Oh, than what [inaudible].

T: Yes.

P: You mean, is that the one I forgot?

T: Yeah. If that's what you'd forgotten. That's what we talked about last time.

P: Of what my image of myself is?

T: Yes. What we agreed on was we were going to look at the **bad** images of yourself.

P: You're saying that if the starting point is defining what the images are now.

T: No, I'm saying that as just history. That's what we agreed last week. That's what you've forgotten.

P: Um.

T: The fact that you've forgotten means either that it was not a good agreement or it wasn't a thorough agreement or was not an agreement, or you just disliked it so much that you forgot it.

P: Well, if we had lots and lots of time I'd love to do that.

T: That's too vague. It's too—too much.

P: Yeah, yeah. Especially with the time limit and and it's, it's uh I don't know it's not [pause] I keep—the word I keep thinking of, it's a trap.

T: Um-hm. I agree with you. It could be just too much room. You tend to run away from things you don't like. Give you too much room . . .

P: Yeah, maybe.

T: You might be able to manage it, to run away all the time.

P: Keep on talking about this and that and being open and honest and still have lots of room to avoid the things. Yeah.

T: Well, there's an experiment that we could try just to see what happened. Which is, we can put three things together and kind of box in an area that's smaller. We can take bad images of yourself—laziness and your brother's death and we can see that just as a miniature experiment for a little bit of time, that we can look into.

P: You mean like try to stick to those [pause]. I, I don't understand.

T: What I mean is that your brother's death really **has** to have meanings for you.

P: Um-hm.

T: It cannot **not** be important.

P: Um-hm.

T: Impossible. You may not have any feelings about it because you're avoiding ideas about it. Your avoiding ideas about it is a kind of laziness.

P: You know I really want to talk about it. I'm really glad that you're talking about it. I'm sitting here saying yes, yes, make me talk about it. I guess I've had enough of putting it off.

T: Yeah. Then that's a bad image of yourself.

P: What? Putting it off?

T: You're a bad person because you've been lazy and putting off realizing the implications of your brother's death.

P: The thing that I was really afraid of, or am, or have toyed with, the idea is that like I think you said it once maybe. There aren't any feelings there.

T: And then you'd be a terrible person.

P: And that's a real fear.

T: And then you'd be a terrible person.

P: Oh, God, yes! [voice gets louder] Here's my favorite brother. And you don't just let your favorite brother die and go, oh yeah. I want to tell you—I'm just bursting with what I want to tell you. I don't know. I had dreamed about him last, this morning um [pause] it was a real nice dream but it wasn't partially I guess 'cause he was alive. And we were saying good-bye because he was going to die. I mean, it was not, you know, a real scary emotional . . . 'cause he was going to go off and kill himself kind of dying. It was like he was going to go away—going on, going on a trip but we were assuring each other that we had always loved each other and wasn't it nice that we had had what we had had. And I said I was going to miss him and he said, "Well, you know there's Gordon. Gordon will be here." I said Gordon is not the same. I don't like Gordon. And he said, "You've never given him a chance." He, I mean he and Gordon were very close, being brothers, and Sam thought the world of him. And he was kind of like saying, "This is my brother." He was kind of giving him to me [pause]. He said, you know, "Give him a chance. There's, he's, he's very deep," or something like that.

T: Yeah.

Note that she brings this dream up late in the hour after the therapist has attempted to refocus.

EIGHTH THERAPY HOUR

By the eighth session, the therapist and patient were able to work together on how she pretended to play roles. For example, the patient had been telling the therapist about a bad episode with Phillip, a subsequent period of depression, but one that had not altered her decision to diet and lose weight. The therapist was relatively supportive in saying, "So that [depressive episode] didn't alter your resolve to diet. You were able to weather that period. And later in the hour, So you're able to say 'No' to yourself." The patient responded verbally to this encouragement but made, at the same time, a face of disparagement. The therapist picked up the nonverbal communication and responded to it.

T: So you're able to say "No" to yourself?
P: Yeah [makes a face]. That's pretty good. I don't know how long it'll last. I, I, I think about it so much in a day.
T: There was that same facial expression again. Yeah! It was somebody else. It's not you.
P: I don't know.
T: I think you're imitating me. I mean not me, really, but some big authority saying something "scientific" to you.
P: Really? Is that a scientifical-looking face?
T: Yeah. Only—yeah, that is.

P: What, what did I just say? [pause] I think it's kind of like a well "well, well, well" face. But it is kind of defecating [she perhaps meant deprecating]. It's kind of like putting yourself down. Looks good on the surface but . . .

T: Underneath its un-

P: . . . yeah, it's like "Okay, go ahead congratulate me for resisting," on Wednesday but I know that it's not going to last or, I know that it wasn't really me that resisted.

T: It's a dumb move to compliment you for resisting because you're really not going to stick to this diet.

P: Yeah. That's it. Yeah.

It was then possible to go from this to an image of herself as manipulator. This was an issue in both the therapeutic relationship (coming under false pretenses) and in the stress event (manipulating siblings to rebel against parents at the funeral, manipulating her own appearance of feelings, such as using tears of anger at her parents as if they were tears of sorrow for her brother).

T: Well, also you think sometimes that you're a bit of a manipulator. See, you ask for attention and then you're afraid when you get it that no one . . .

P: Really meant it.

T: . . . gave it to you because it's **interesting** to give you attention; that they just gave it to you because you're such a **needy** person or something.

P: Um-hm. Um-hm.

T: Someone shows admiration for something you do and you think you've conned them into it. You don't feel you really deserved it. I think you have a lot of doubts about what you do deserve.

P: [Long pause] I will put myself in a double bind doing that, too, because I ask—I get mad if I don't get compliments. But I can't accept them when I do get them, 'cause I feel that I've asked for them, in one way or another. [long pause]. I don't feel like I deserve to be loved. You know, like I'm just wandering around after Phillip or whoever and saying, "Love me, love me, love me." I don't really expect that, [for them] to turn around and love me.

T: Well, even when you were asking him to be nice to you it did have a somewhat hostile quality, didn't it? Of nagging him to love you?

P: Um-hm. Well, I'm aware of it while I'm doing it.

T: Yeah.

P: Um.

T: You're not exactly saying, "There, I am ready to be loved. Here I am lovable. I'm loving you, ready to be loved in return." You're saying, "You see, you don't love me." You just tone it down a little so that it's a little obscure.

P: I say, "You see, you don't love me," but I also say, "Here I am, **unlovable**."

T: Yeah.

P: "I want you to love me, anyway, but you're a jerk if you do." Uh. And, "I don't believe you if you say you do." Um. "You may be thinking it now, but you're not going to tomorrow," that kind of thing [long pause].

EIGHTH THROUGH ELEVENTH THERAPY HOURS

In hours 8 through 11 the therapeutic alliance was established, and it was used as an umbrella of trust under which the homesickness–funeral constellation was worked through. This work will be discussed in Appendix B, beginning with its precursors in earlier hours. This section of therapy dealt with the relatively difficult task, as compared with the average therapy, of establishing a therapeutic alliance. Toward the end of the final treatment hour Janice emphasized the importance of this work earlier in the treatment.

P: . . . What I've doubted was you.
T: Yeah?
P: Whether you could, uh, do it, whether you could [pause] understand what I was saying and not take sides and, uh, [pause] make me work, kind of, make me go further than what I could do by myself. Be objective. You know just do all the things that you're supposed to do and—[pause]. And I wasn't at all sure what to do [pause]. It's like I could have, I would have known if you had been doing just a formula or, or your impersonation of a shrink or something like that or you had been coming at me from a theory. Like, um [pause]. I don't feel, I don't feel like you've tried to put a definition on me.

POSTTHERAPY EVALUATION INTERVIEW

Further information on the importance to her of the therapeutic alliance is found in the follow-up evaluation interview, conducted by another clinician months after the final treatment interview.

E (Evaluator): Where did you feel that Dr. Jones was, on that judgmental listening and accepting scale? Where would you put him?
P: Oh, I thought he was terrific. It felt good. At first I was frustrated because I wanted him to be a little more judgmental and . . . on my side, like to take up arms about my supervisor, like that. But, then I realized that it was really a relief that h . . . for him to be as objective as he was because, I didn't have to play games. I didn't have to try to keep up a good impression and, um, and I didn't feel that he had a bad impression I had to overcome by dazzling him or anything.
E: So, it was okay to be yourself a . . .
P: So, yeah, right, so I could say just about anything.

She also reported her memory of difficulties in establishing a focus for therapeutic communication.

E: What do you remember about what your original contract was with him?

P: You know, I forgot in the middle of the session what the original contract was. We dealt with that one time. I talked to him and I said I don't remember. He tried to help me remember. After saying that, I still couldn't remember. What I wanted him to say, what I wanted the contract to be was—help me find out about these areas that I don't like in myself and what I can do about them. And then we, at least, if you can't cure me set me on the path and what he, he . . .

E: So the focus that you had in mind was really your whole life, then.

P: Yeah, my whole life and, and uh, setting me on the road to the whole life that I wanted. And I, I don't remember the first ways he phrased it. Eventually, we, um, what laziness was the key word and we decided to talk about my bad feelings, and, of course, he very carefully got into bad feelings that I had about myself and using laziness as, like a central issue.

E: How much were your feelings about your brother a part of the original contract?

P: They were more a part of the original contract than they were of my understanding of it, and, and of my remembrance of the revised one.

E: Oh, so the contract got revised along the way then.

P: I think so. Um, as soon as he told me that we didn't have to talk about my brother, and I spent a lot of time feeling guilty 'cause I was in here wanting to talk about my whole life and not really aware of feeling all that shook up about my brother and hearing this crisis thing [criterion of the stress clinic] and I didn't want to talk about the crisis. But as soon as he let me know that we didn't have to talk about the crisis and we could talk about different parts of my life and anything like that, um, I found, once or twice, I found myself wanting to talk about my brother.

E: So, when he said it was okay not to, then some of the feelings for your brother came up.

P: Um-hm. I remember coming in one time and telling him about a dream and stuff—and even then he didn't like, I guess I was waiting for him to pounce and say, "Aha! The meat of the matter! Let's get down to talking about what you really came here for!" He just calmly talked about it, and I don't think we even spent the whole time on it.

E: So you didn't feel pushed that there was only one area that it was okay to talk about then.

In the third evaluation interview, conducted 11 months after the termination of therapy, she again reported her view of the therapeutic alliance. She said, "I really liked Dr. Jones's objectivity. I, I felt myself being able to just be myself. Instead of like trying to impress him or trying to win his sympathy or anything."

SUMMARY

An important test of the therapeutic possibilities of the relationship was to see if she could fool the therapist about two issues. One was that she was self-sufficient, the other was that she would cry over her brother if the therapist did the right thing. If she **fooled** the therapist into thinking she was self-sufficient, she could stabilize herself in the pretending *tra-la-la* state. But the disadvantage was that she would not get help and would continue to be depressed. If she did **not fool** the therapist into thinking that she was self-sufficient, she could then hope that the therapist would be able to help her despite herself. But then there was the threat that she might feel humiliated, expect criticism, and enter the *self-disgusted* state.

Similar problems were involved over the idea that the therapy was to help her cry about the death of her brother. If she succeeded in fooling the therapist into thinking that, then he might help her cry over her brother. That would help her avoid images of self-disgust, but risked her contempt of the therapist because he went along with a mistaken idea because it suited him. If, as she really hoped, the therapist was not fooled into thinking she had come only to cry over her brother, then she could hope the therapy would work. But with that hope came the fear of accusations that she came under false pretenses, and fear of rejection if she did not match up to the special interests of the clinic and the therapist. The therapeutic alliance was a protection against all these dangers. Reduction of relationship dangers and the presence of the real relationship allowed her to work on other issues. Her separation conflicts and her reactions to the death and funeral were one manifestation of this developmental crisis. This constellation has been called the home-sickness theme, and segments of the therapy excerpted according to such topics are presented in Appendix B.

B.   WORKING THROUGH: THE HOMESICKNESS THEME

The homesickness theme is a complex constellation, as described in Chapters 4 and 7. It involves the following conflicting elements: (1) a wish to separate herself from her mother and become independent and autonomous, (2) self-criticism that she had not completed this life task, (3) fear and guilt that leaving would hurt her mother, (4) resentment that her mother did not permit her to go her own way but urged Janice to stay with her and be like her, (5) criticism of her mother for being the wrong kind of person with whom to identify, (6) longing to join forces with her mother, (7) hostility and criticism of her mother for not loving her more, (8) a sense of self-injury as a result of the loss of her brother, who functioned in part to stabilize her sense of identity as independent from her mother, (9) sadness over the loss of her brother with a complementary fear of being lost as he was, and (10) remorse that at his funeral she had behaved inappropriately out of a regressive rebellion against her mother and father. At the beginning of treatment, these themes were not faced squarely by the patient. They were communicated to the therapist in fragments, with a variety of avoidances and distortions when threatening ideas and feelings emerged. Here the process of identification of these themes and a partial working through will be illustrated by additional excerpts from the therapy transcripts.

EVALUATION BEFORE THERAPY

The importance of Janice's relationship to her mother, as symbolized and reactivated by her brother's funeral, was mentioned in passing during the first evaluation session.

P: So it's with Mom that we can have most of our dealings, especially me being the daughter and all, and we share a lot of [pause] confidence. My mother thinks I'm a slut and a nymphomaniac, and that I'll never be happy because I've ruined my life.

This type of switching of attitudes, and alternating positive and negative role models was a typical maneuver of undoing, as described in Chapter 4. She went on to speak briefly about the funeral.

P: When I went home I really upset my mother because I kept going upstairs and reading. And, you know, she says, "You're here. We want to see you. Can't you sit down and read with us?" Well, that's not the point. I wanted to get away. I don't think I said that to her, I tried to explain it to her, "Mom, this is **my** way of dealing with it."

FIRST THERAPY HOUR

In the first hour of treatment, she brought up the theme of homesickness but in a disavowed form. She said she did not miss another person, a woman friend who instead missed her. This woman friend may also symbolize her mother, who misses her and wants her home. She followed this by a statement disavowing homesickness.

P: Really, that I don't miss her. She misses me a lot [pause]. And I wonder if it's because the minute she's not there if I've got to kind of make her unreal. I put her in a timeless slot, and I expect her to stay the same. And, you know, like, I can take her out of a drawer.
T: Yeah.
P: But it's the same with my family, I don't get homesick.
T: Yeah.
P: I hardly ever get [pause] every once in a while.

As she spoke, she heard what she said as if with the objective ears of the therapist. In midstatement she corrected herself from what would have been "I hardly ever get homesick" to "Every once in a while I get homesick." The therapist noted such clues, as reflected in his process notes.

SECOND THERAPY HOUR

This theme emerged again in the second therapy hour. She said she had been worried about losing Phillip because he might have a brain tumor. The only sign of this was an occasional slurring of his speech. The therapist thought this could be a displaced fear of repetition of the loss of her brother. She denied any feelings about her brother and her separation from her family. The therapist was relatively quiet, saying "Uh-huh" and "Yes" occasionally.

After a long pause she then said, "I [pause] did I tell you that I never get homesick? That I don't miss my family and I don't miss my friends? And I keep trying to find a theory to explain it, that's allowable [pause]. Why don't I miss them? Well, because I know they're there and I know they love me and they're always with me in my heart or something like that. I think what it is, is that the minute anybody's gone from my sight they become a person in a book that I'm fond of."

FIFTH THERAPY HOUR

The homesickness issue did not emerge in the third and fourth hours, which centered on issues of the therapeutic alliance. It did surface again in the fifth hour. She talked about accepting or rejecting her mother's definition of her and about identifying or not identifying with her mother. The thrapist missed the center of the theme and instead focused a little off center on attitudes about sexual freedom, probably recalling an earlier statement where she mentioned that her mother had called her a nymphomaniac. This error of focus was then corrected by the therapist.

T: Modern [repeating a word she has used about her type of woman]?

P: Modern? I mean, like, uh [pause] I might have found it easier to accept my mother's definition [pause] than [pause], then [pause] the one [pause] woman that I want to be, you know, just to [pause] just to, uh, go to college, work for two years, get married, have children [pause] uh [pause]. You know, the question never [pause] anything never [pause] you know, that's it, that's success. Then what you worry about is being a good mother, and you torture yourself because of whether you're ruining your children or something like that. But— [pause].

T: I have a feeling that hovering not too far out of your consciousness is your sexual freedom, and that you're too embarrassed to bring it up [long pause].

P: Maybe. Although hearing you say that twice after I've avoided it makes me feel like, oh, wow, it's really . . . All right, we can talk about sex. Okay, maybe it is [a problem, or embarrassing], and I'm not aware of it. [She is telling the therapist she is not upset about sexuality.]

T: No. Well, then I'm wrong because what I was suggesting was that you were aware of something and not telling me, and I was wrong about that.

P: Um [pause] um [pause] I've always been amazed at how well-adjusted sexually I seem to be.

T: M-hm.

P: Because I should have been completely screwed up because of my parents' attitudes and . . . and . . . then because of some of the changes I went through.

T: Yeah, their attitudes. They seem quite critical of your living with somebody.

P: Oh, "It's horrible." I . . . I [laughs] "threw away my virginity" [pause]. . . . And my mother found out and was stricken, and that's about when she started the "You-used-to-be-so-sweet-and-thoughtful" routine. "You used to be so wonderful, how could you have changed?"

T: Huh.

P: And she was amazed that I had been living in the house and acting the same when all this had been going on.

T: So I hear that that's a very debased self-image projected on you by your mother.

P: Uh-huh. The thing that I felt, though, that I finally realized that I felt at that time, was anger at her for acting that way, because I had been punishing myself through the whole relationship by feeling guilty, by being worried about being pregnant, by being worried about being caught, by being worried that he didn't really love me, which was true, and . . . and all this stuff. And as soon as she was found . . . as soon as I was found out, it was over. Whew! That's over. And I had already paid as far as I was concerned. And she went on and on and on, punishing me. And in a way she still is.

T: Hm.

P: Hm.

T: Your mother has a bad image of you.

P: Oh, yeah.

T: And it rankles you.

P: Drives me crazy [pause]. Well, after that I [pause] I didn't really feel much guilt [long pause]. I've been lucky. I think I've been purposely naive a lot [pause]. And that saved me from being hurt on a lot of occasions.

T: You kind of protect yourself by . . .

P: Un-huh.

T: . . . By not knowing.

P: Uh-huh.

Here the therapist failed to clarify the issue adequately. He focused on the mother's bad image of her, instead of her reciprocal bad image of her mother and, therefore, the bad image she had of herself if she thought of being like her mother.

Later in this hour she talked about how she read for long periods of time and withdrew from social contacts. The therapist told her that she did this to reduce her anxiety and loneliness. After she responded he interpreted her homesickness directly.

P: Uh-huh. Why would a . . . [long pause]. It seems funny to say, lonely. I can't quite agree, but I can't disagree [pause]. In some ways I had a really, really happy childhood.

T: Yeah. That's why I find it funny that I find myself using that word, yet you come across to me as being lonely.

P: Hm [pause].

T: I have a feeling that you're homesick.

P: Do you remember that hot weather? [pause] Um, what was it, a week and a half ago?

T: Yeah.

P: I got **so** homesick and that's the first time, really, since being out here. I've had one or two flashes, once when it rained I thought of our house by the lake and I wanted to be there. But that hot weather . . [pause] in the summer is really hot and muggy, and [pause] I was really homesick. And it wasn't for the people, as they are now, it was for my childhood. I wanted to be at the lake. I wanted to go hiking with my brothers [pause], you know, to fish [pause] sit in the living room and listen to the rocking chair creak, and somebody making tea, and **everything!**

T: Uh-huh. Well, it sounds nice.

P: **Oh**, it's really, that's, that's my home, by the lake.

SIXTH THERAPY HOUR

The theme of homesickness is now somewhat more available to Janice than it was, earlier. She began the next hour, session six, by asking the therapist for help with her stomach pains. This was more than a simple request, it tested the relationship to see if the therapist would maintain the therapeutic alliance or comply with the role model of potential transference by accepting the position of rescuer. The therapist expressed an interest in hearing about the stomach pains but did not accept responsibility for diagnosing or treating them.

She then asked for help with how to handle an argument with Phillip. She talked about how she wanted Phillip to reassure her all the time. The therapist told her that she spoke of wanting to move out but was unwilling to think through this issue because she was afraid to contemplate being alone. She went on to say that she was disgusted with herself for poisoning every relationship she touched. She described herself as having sucked and sucked from other persons, as being lazy and selfish when it came to giving in to their needs. She compared herself to a vampire and told about how frightened she was at a recent vampire movie. She then described the reverse role relationship, her fear that Phillip would leave her in a depleted state.

SEVENTH THERAPY HOUR

In the seventh session she expressed confusion about the aim of the therapy. The therapist reminded her of the termination and her agreement to focus on her self-criticisms. She then described the dream about her dead brother in which they were going to separate (material excerpted in Appendix A). In the dream her brother was going on a long trip, but reassured her that they had always loved each other and she would still have her other brother. In discussing the brother, she compared herself to her mother in an abstract way. The mother also was sitting around crying because her dead son was not there to give her hugs. The therapist then asked her to consciously use her often unconscious defense, avoidance of emotion, and intellectual exploration of ideas. The following excerpt was microanalyzed in Chapter 7.

T: But let's be . . . let's be very rational, very intellectual about it. What does
     it really mean to you that Sam is dead? [pause] In terms of you? What does
     it. . . .

P: My life?

T: What does . . . what meanings does it have? Be very reasonable.

P: Well, nothing in . . . in terms of the things like coming in and giving hugs and stuff it's [pause] it means the occasional letter that isn't there, the admiration that he had for me. That asking for big-sisterly advice kind of thing [long pause]. It means I don't like the mention of anything about it [long pause]. Um. I don't know, doesn't mean, doesn't mean anything that I can put my finger on.

T: Yeah, you know, we just took that level and it doesn't have any big implications for your life on that level at all.

Here again the therapist uses a maneuver he has found effective with her. He makes an extreme statement at one pole of the oscillation between "it does" and "it doesn't." She then asserts the obverse pole more insistently and distinctly.

P: In a way it does, 'cause it [pause] it really brings home the unreality of things. And, like, he was **there** on faith. I hadn't seen him for a year, but I knew he was there. I had the faith. I believed he was there. And now he's **not** there, and I have to take **that** on faith, too. [Sniffles] I'm so, uh [pause] what's real and what isn't? Is anybody else there? Now, all these people that I remember, that I feel close to, that I have this faith in [pause], maybe they're not real either.

T: Yeah. Well, it symbolizes, then, a larger realm of meanings, which is that the family whom you were attached to, your childhood and adolescent family, is no longer **there** for you, because you're no longer a child or an adolescent. **You've** become independent.

Note that the therapist took a definite position. By saying that she had already become independent he said, in effect, that she was not homesick. She could then show strength by opposing him, to counterbalance expressing a "weakness." She went on to say that she was homesick, by saying, "When I get homesick":

P: When I get homesick, I get homesick for childhood things and places. It's [pause] it's not a now, a present-day homesickness. It's not like I physically need, physically want to go back there and do what's going on now, or I'd live there now. I want to go back in time, too [long pause].

T: Sure. Then you had some pretty reliable ties to people. Your ties with Phillip aren't so reliable [pause].

P: No, not at all.

EIGHTH THERAPY HOUR

She went back and forth modulating expression of just how home-sick she was. She said it, denied or qualified it, then asserted it most clearly as "I want to go back in time." The therapist linked the issue to what she had been talking about, her current difficulties with Phillip.

This marks an important point in the therapy. She reported states of *crying* after the session. In the next hour she worked more intensely than previously. This began the phase of working through that lasted through the eleventh session. Here is an excerpt from the early part of that eighth session:

P: I had, uh, a bad day this week, uh, Tuesday [the day of her previous session]. [Pause] or Wednesday. Um. I got my period early this month, and I've been on a different kind of pill this month but [trails off] on Wednesday I had another weepy day, and spent the whole day crying about everything and anything and nothing. Usuallly, if somebody says, "Go ahead and cry," I can't. I dry out, and I'll [pause] be damned if I'm going to cry 'cause they said it's all right. But Phillip said, "Go ahead and cry." And [I] went ahead and cried. Didn't even have to think of anything sad. Okay, "boo hoo." And it started to bother me about halfway through the afternoon because I was really bothering him, dripping around all afternoon and he was patting me on the head. So [pause] and, uh, I started saying, "Why am I doing this? What's happening? I don't know why this is." But at the same time I didn't feel the, uh [pause] despair that I felt when that's happened before. And it's frightening because I don't know why this is. But at the same time I didn't feel the, uh [pause] I didn't know why. And it does seem, uh, like I'm out of control and everything. And I also have this feeling that it's connected with every other time I've been depressed. That [pause] that [pause] it's like [pause] a subterranean lake or something. And there's all these wells that go down to it. And, and most of the time I'm walking on the surface, but every once in a while I, I extend down toward the wells and get in touch with this great big lake of depression.

T: M-hm.

P: Which is always the same, always has been and always will be this feeling permanence and nothing. That never changes, it's always there underneath. And the feeling, I really get into that. I don't know if that's coincidental or not.

T: Well, there's one thing that can't be coincidental, which is when you have that, when you get in touch with that feeling, you want to attach yourself to somebody. So you went to following Phillip around, wanting some kind of, uh, supplies from him.

P: M-hm.

T: And that would have to sort of, I would think, have to relate in some way to you having left home just about a year ago. That is, you want to school for four years and that was a kind of . . .

P: Well, in my hometown [sarcastically], I mean—

T: [Interrupts] Interim, yeah, but now there you are still . . .

P: Gung ho for the Sundays.

T: Yeah. And, uh, then you left home about a year ago. You had these feelings of kind of anguish at times which you've never been specific about. You've never felt specifically homesick from what you've said.

P: Um. Uh-uhm [pause]. No. I know that I want something badly, and I want love and security, comfort, things like that [pause]. I think if I can verbalize that and ask for attention and physical comforting, reassurance and stuff . . . [pause].

T: I don't know if you can. I know you do, but maybe you do it kind of dramatically. At least you describe it that—

P: [Interrupts enthusiastically] I do it dramatically and I do it crookedly. I do it sideways as long as I can. Skirt around, like, when I wanted him to say that he loved me. I couldn't come right out and say, "Tell me that you love me." One thing, what if he didn't? For another, when, you ask, it's not as good as if he had just done it by himself. Um [pause] I went around and around and around the issue. Please do this, please do that. If he didn't do exactly what I wanted it gave me fits. I guess him doing what I want would be loving me. And I asked him for . . . for, uh, hugs, and I asked him for kisses, and I finally asked him to tell me something nice. And he couldn't even manage to say that it was a nice day.

Later, the therapist said, "I think you have a great yearning to plug into somebody." She responded, "Oh, I think that's true, and I think that's part of the reason why I went around talking [about her brother's death] to everyone before, you know, and saying things over and over again to different people, hoping maybe there'd be a spark somewhere." As an indication of the kind of cooperative therapeutic work that was now possible, here is an excerpt from later in this eighth interview:

T: And, really, by asking you to come home they're [her parents] in a way criticizing you. They're saying, "Well, you're not going to do it" [become independent].

P: "You didn't do it." Yeah.

T: "You just admit that you failed and come on back home to the nest."

P: "We'll talk to somebody we know and get you a nice job."

T: "You'll never have to leave home, you'll never have to grow up. And we'll all be one big happy family. But you have to admit that you failed."

P: M-hm.

T: In order to crawl back [pause].

P: I don't have images of, uh, I should start fantasizing on that . . . on that as being a success and going home and telling them off. I guess I have been showing them all 'cause I **haven't** been coming home. You know, the fantasy is pulling up to the door, in a great big Lear jet. Why not?

T: Sure. It's a fantasy, you might as well.

P: [Laughs] I can just see it sitting on the street.

T: But it's true, you don't. I have not heard from you in any way, any fantasies of that kind of . . .

P: Or anything like that, no. Part . . . part of it is probably because I haven't got the faintest idea of what they really want. I . . . I don't know if I know exactly what they want from me. I don't think that having what I would define as a good job would be enough. Yeah.

T: What would you have to do, become president?

P: Um, they'd probably still be able to. . . .

T: Write the Bible?

P: Write the **Bible** would probably do it [laughs].

T: Really.

P: They'd probably still be able to, uh, have reservations, even if I was president cause they'd wonder if I were really happy. This is the thing, that's what my mother says, "You can't be really happy leading the kind of life you are."

T: There's a certain amount of hostility in that interaction.

P: M-hm. Oh, well. She obviously doesn't approve of the kind of life I lead.

T: Her saying that makes you feel badly.

P: M-hm [pause]. I think one of the reasons that I have so many high images that I keep trying to live up to is that I spent so long trying to please them, trying to get their approval.

NINTH THERAPY HOUR

In the next hour, the ninth, the therapist is able to confront her again with distancing herself from a real confrontation with her present position. Here is an excerpt from that session:

T: I have a feeling, you're moving away from me. I don't really have a clear picture of this at all, where you stand on what you're doing and what you want to do. It just doesn't make enough sense to me somehow, which is why I feel you're not, not making it clear to me and [trails off].

The therapist took a position for her. He was not seeing things clearly, just as she was not experiencing the theme directly, but rather in a mildly depersonalized way. He repeated the challenge that she make him understand, in an effort to have her express herself directly enough so that she too would understand. Sharing the need to understand would help to accomplish this. The manner of the therapist was incisive so that she could share his sense of confidence in her ability to confront and integrate the ideas and feelings. She struggled with this, became exasperated, and had a "strong" self-image to counteract the danger of emergence of her weak, dejected, and "disgusting" self-image.

P: Well, it's 'cause it's not clear to me. You see, because I'm not thinking about what is this for, where am I going, uh, what I'm doing is not working.

T: [Incisively] You're **not** working and you're **not** going to get married to Phillip, and that's about where you're **at**. And, uh,. . . .

P: [More argumentative] I'm waiting, I'm waiting for Bob and Carol to come out.

T: [Sarcastic] Yeah, and they're bringing a fortune cookie with the answer to it in there?

P: [Subdued, earnest, reflective] Maybe. Yeah. They're bringing me . . . [pause] . . . they're bringing a me that I like. They both **love** me.

T: M-hm.

P: And they let me know it.

T: Yeah.

P: And they've known me for about ten years or more [pause]. And I'm really counting on having their support and having them to bounce myself off of.

T: [Incisive] Yeah, but what about **me**? Why am **I** in the dark now? Why am I feeling that I don't know what's going on with you? [Pause.]

P: I don't know. I don't feel that I'm trying to hide anything from you, particularly.

T: M-hm.

P: It's probably just cause I don't . . .

T: [Earnestly] I thought maybe you were sharing that feeling though.

P: Like what, that I don't know what's going on?

T: Yeah.

P: [Somewhat petulantly] Well, I just don't want to **think** about it. I don't **want to** think, "Where am I going?" or "What am I doing?"

T: [Firmly] Yeah, but what would you think of **me** if I let you get away with that?

The therapist placed the construct of "laziness" upon himself as he asked for the patient's attitude if he were to procrastinate and not confront her with the next issues in her life, and let the therapy "run out." By externalization of the particular image, her reactions to it could be sharpened. She was also being asked to perform a process consciously, to externalize meanings, one that she usually performed unconsciously.

P: No, I mean that's probably why **you** feel hazy is because **I'm** being purposely hazy to myself.

T: [Firmly] Yeah, but what will you think of me if I don't, uh, say anything about that, if I just let it just roll on like that?

P: You're probably as fuzzy as I am.

T: We have a limited amount of time left. We have to finish by the end of the month. What if I just didn't, uh, say any, if I kept silent about that? **I mean it**, what would you think of me?

P: [Pause] I'm not sure.

T: Would it be **okay** with you if I did not say anything else about that?

P: I might not even notice, probably underneath. But see, I'm not even sure what . . . what it is that you're keeping silent about, and I, I'm getting very confused, too.

T: M-hm. Oh.

P: [Very vague] Um, if you didn't think anything about your confusion about where I am and what I'm doing right now.

T: Yeah, yeah. I guess it would be a version of laziness, [pause] or whatever we're calling laziness, whatever. That's probably a pseudolaziness, whatever it is.

P: I don't know if that is what I'm doing. It's [becomes incisive] it's fear and laziness. I don't want to think. I want to take the whole summer off. I don't want to . . . I don't want to [pause] do much more than what I'm doing with you. I don't want to think about, uh [pause] going to school, "Am I early enough?" I don't want to think about the fall. "Do I really want that job back again?" If not, "what else?" I don't want to think about the kind of the person that I want to be.

The patient is being firm, now, like the therapist, and expects the therapist to be satisfied with this, because she has been a "good student" and has said something the "teacher" wants to hear. But the therapist decides to press the issue even further.

T: Yes, but the question is, What will you think of **me** if **I** go **on** with that position? I'll say, "Well, we only had a few more, July, it's just a month. I don't want to . . . I want to take . . . I don't want to deal with her—"

P: [Interrupts] I've got . . . I mean—

T: [Overriding her] I don't want to deal with her. I don't want to deal with her in that way.

P: [Petulant and a little angry] Um, I'd probably stop coming. [Pause] If that was your attitude, I mean if it came through to me that way that you didn't press certain issues because "well, we only have so much time and, after all, we can stick to the easy ones." 'Cause, I, um, that would make me feel . . . rejected.

T: Mm.

P: And, um, uninteresting, **unimportant**. "Well, if it's not, not worth it to him, then I'm certainly not going to, you know, go through the motions."

T: Yeah.

A short while later there is a focus directly on the homesickness theme. The therapist now took a softer, more supportive role, allowing her to take a critical position.

T: [Acceptingly] Maybe you feel you deserve a vacation. You've been functioning on your own for almost a year [pause]. You don't want that to be hard for you but [trails off].

P: [Assertively] I don't. I really don't and I hate to think that that's it, that it's just that I'm on my own now and I don't have my parents and my hometown.

T: [Softly] Well, it's the first year for you.

P: It is. But that doesn't count.

She then went on to give much more detail about her current history, about her feelings when she left home, what had happened until now, and how she sometimes felt that her parents did not love her.

TENTH THERAPY HOUR

In the next hour she said she had been feeling better and better and had more of a sense of where she wanted to go. She talked about how she had looked through a scrapbook where there were pictures of her brother, and had felt choked up for the first time. She felt she could really cry now if she let herself, and it would be authentic. This led her to recount the visit home for the funeral.

The therapist asked her to go back in her mind to these memories, an effort at abreaction. This led to a description of the difficulties with her mother and her own behavior patterns during the funeral. She related their mutual anger, especially that of her mother, who scolded her for being irreverent and silly, for joking at various times, withdrawing to her room and not being with the family. She also related how she used her tears of anger with her mother to pretend she was crying about Sam.

T: Would you go back in your memory to when you went home after Sam's death and you were with the family? Let's go back to that point in time in your memory. See what thoughts you find in your mind then. Relate it to this issue: They're showing a lot of grief and you're not showing any and what should you be doing?

P: My mother even said to me that she wished I wouldn't go upstairs and read all the time, but at **least** I could come down and read with friends. But the implication is that [mumbles something about that she could be with family, that this is a time to be together] [pause]. And I felt bad about that but also kind of defiant, and, "Mom, this is what I need to do, and I don't have to be running upstairs all the time with a book and some food" [pause]. And, um [pause].

T: What were you running from? You're not running from reactions to Sam's death at that point. I don't believe that [pause]. It doesn't hang together well enough. It must be something else, I think.

P: You don't think it's because maybe I would have to [mumbles something about having sad feelings].

T: Well, maybe. But I don't believe it right now. Let's just. . . .

P: That's what I thought that it was. That everything I didn't want to deal with . . .

T: I think you didn't want to deal with your family.

P: Yeah. I think that's very true [long pause]. I didn't want to have to talk with them. I didn't want to have to be comforted by them [pause]. I remember crying one night, a night or two after I came home, getting **really mad** at my mother and going upstairs and starting to cry out of anger and then using the already crying to try to cry about Sam a little bit and feeling better.

T: I'd like to hear about the anger with your mother.

P: She bawled me out! We had just met at the airport, and we had been joking, joking all the way from the airport.It was one of those kind of things where we all got together and got silly. And it was a real relief sort of thing. And Mom was being very disapproving, pursing her lips. I kept on practically challenging her to say, "You're being irreverent."

Since she seemed to do well under the therapeutic alliance, with the therapist pushing her gently toward verbalizing her feelings, he continued this nuance. Here is one excerpt from that type of work:

P: I have to be a hypocrite and still follow along, and act the way my mom thinks we should be. She'd warn me and she said, "Please don't act like that in church."

T: Which isn't for Sam. It's for the family's appearances.

P: [Inaudible segment] And, um, I poured it all off on the next day. Very bitterly and I felt guilty at the time for doing it, like, I was getting back at Mom by getting support from the others.

T: You were angry at your mother.

P: I just really was, yeah.

T: Your mother was angry at you.

P: And [pause].

T: Your mother was criticizing you.

P: She was criticizing me, and, and she was also doing it real heavily, because like I said, "This is a time when a family should support each other," and "We're supposed to all be really together." And, and, and, couldn't I come through even just this once kind of thing.

T: Just this once.

P: Well, it's not like I never do. I heard that, and it didn't sound right as soon as I said it; but that was the kind of feeling I got.

T: It shows how **bad** you are.

P: Yeah.

T: You were a **very bad girl**.

P: Um-hm. And, and, and . . .

T: You agree with that at some level. You feel you were a very bad girl. You were. You were, uh, leading your brothers and sisters down the path of silliness. And, now, you have to make up for it by having a big . . .

P: Trauma?

T: Big trauma [pause].

P: I don't know, it seems kind of a little farfetched [pause]. Partially, well, I don't know. If I were letting her know that I were being traumatized I would agree more. "Look, Mom, look how I'm suffering" [pause]. And in a way I'd **like** her to know. I'm mad at her right now because she never asks how I am.

T: Oh.

P: You know, in letters and stuff. I mean maybe conventionally, "Hi, how are you?" "I'm fine." That kind of stuff. But she never [pause] I don't know, I want her to sense that there's something wrong, and I want her to ask about it [pause]. I said to her one time, before I came, I think, before I started seeing you, I told her that I had been crying that afternoon, and I couldn't really realize that he was gone and that I felt weepy a lot and she said she and my sister did, too. And it was a bond kind of thing. I said the right thing and she said the right thing back.

There is then a restatement of themes that emerged earlier in the hour.

T: Yeah. You liked the idea of yourself crying [at the funeral]. You clearly felt guilty that you weren't crying.

P: M-hm.

T:. Whenever you could cry about something, you'd have liked it to be seen by the people.

P: Well [pause], definitely I felt it that time, and I **was** really glad that everybody saw it.

T: You were feeling badly about the way you were, which was angry and disgusted and withdrawn.

P: M-hm.

T: And you were also feeling anxious about being sucked in somehow. I mean I think there must have been some anxiety that you would do just what your mother wanted you to do. You'd fold yourself up in her arms like Mrs. Smith.

P: [Long pause] And I kept being tempted to do that, too. Um, came off the plane with my lip-trembling kind of thing and at various times I could have [pause] fallen on her breast with tears and wailed. I wouldn't even have had to do that. I am definitely afraid of drama because I know I like it, and it's just that it, it's not [trails off].

T: Well, it ran rightfully so.

P: What do you mean?

T: Well, this isn't the time in your life to go back to your mother's bosom.

P: M-hm. But I, I could have just gotten a little amount of approval [pause] by breaking down and crying at certain points but I didn't. Or by not being silly.

T: Mm. No, I think you were feeling maybe unconsciously, that that's kind of dangerous, being sucked in.

P: Like, I went out of my way not to.

T: You went out of your way, yeah.

P: That really makes sense because I can see her just wanting me to stay there, you know, not to go back to California. "Stay here, we need you now." Um, in fact, I was really angry when I heard that Bob had said to Carol, his roommate who is also a friend of mine, that he wouldn't be surprised if I came back.

T: Mm.

P: And I went, "What! I thought you knew me better than that!" And on and on and on [makes sounds of outrage].

ELEVENTH THERAPY HOUR

   In the 11th hour, the next to the last, she picked up the theme again and said it had been on her mind since the previous hour. She kept thinking about her parents, especially about not knowing what they were really like. At the same time she felt that they wanted her to be a carbon copy of her mother. She realized she had always rebelled against that, especially in high school. Becoming a part of a peer "hippy" group had not felt authentic either. She was a misfit, was not suited to either the mold of convention or that of a counteridentity group. She then said, "I couldn't play any of the right roles because I didn't want to be sucked in. And I think that's been really, really true at least the last year and maybe longer. As though I was trying desperately not to [pause] stay home, or go home, or [pause] feel at home, I don't think. And it's something I'm really afraid of . . ." [pause].

She continued, "I feel so strongly about it. I was walking down the street the other day, thinking about what we've been talking about, and once again I feel indignation at my friend for suggesting that I might stay at home [at the time of the funeral and because of the death], feeling what I felt then. It was like, you know, heh, could I ever. I couldn't possibly! No way could I ever! I mean I couldn't possibly! And, like, no matter what happened, no matter if I had no one else in the city that I knew, I probably could have come back here because it's just barely far enough away [from her parents]." She then carries forward this determination not to return home as she says, "I mean none of these things that my mother does to try to make me come home all the time. I mean, 'We'll pay your transportation, you can live with us,' that doesn't affect me at all." The therapist said, "You would **like** to be able to say that."

She continued talking about how her mother tried to make her come home. In addition to being real, this statement typified her externalization of her own regressive wish to return home. To support the stronger counterwish to continue her independent development, the therapist then asked, "How do you envision the future?" This was an effort to carry her forward to a train of thought in which she would develop plans, tolerate the anxiety of not knowing what her plans were for sure, but develop hope that she could consciously set independent goals and then deliberately accomplish them and feel intact and adult.

Her answer to the question was "The immediate—like within a year or two, or the distant future?" This was an effort to get the therapist to supply more direction and to avoid having to answer the question. The therapist answered with only one word, "immediate." The defensive nature of the question was then seen again in her response: "I can leap over a few years and have it all mapped out. It's just the next few years, I don't, I just [trails off and pauses]." The therapist again focused attention on the subject by this clarification: "I think it's the next two or three steps that are very fuzzy." She said "Uh-huh [pause] sure." She went on to talk about her plans about going to school and moving out of her apartment, a reference to the issue of whether or not to break with Phillip.

After dealing with future plans the therapist then highlighted one issue for her. She talked about the future plans in the light of what her parents expected her to do and not in terms of her own wishes. He then said "Well, would it embarrass you if you were to find out that you wanted your mother's approval of you?" She responded by focusing on the relationship between herself and her mother.

P: I don't know. I don't think so because I know I really do. I know that it really, really hurts me that she doesn't give it and I keep trying for it. I, I do things like uh, I get really hurt when I do something to please her and she's not pleased enough. Or when I do something to please her and she's pleased about the thing but she brings in all her qualifiers. Like "Yes dear, it's nice that you did such and such. But why can't you . . . [pause] leave Phillip . . . or come home or straighten up or whatever. Yes, we're glad that you got a job finally."

    She's never pleased enough. She, you know, I called her up all excited. "Mom, Mom. I got a job. And it's going to be so neat. I'm going to get to use my skills and I'm going to get paid a decent amount and I only work six hours and I like it and on and on and on. And she'll say kind of like "Oh, how nice" [pause]. Um—"Does it mean you can move?" [away from Phillip] And that's, that's all it meant to her and [pause] and I really expected her to be more pleased. I expected it to be the kind of job she would approve of. In fact I thought, I guess I thought it was a nice compromise. Something that I could like and be myself in and something that would please every-body else too [sniff, pause].

T: Yeah, I could see how that would hurt your feelings.

P: Um-hm, it did.

T: And I can see how being a proud person, you wouldn't want to know that.

P: What, that it hurt my feelings?

T: Yeah.

P: Maybe. I don't sit around thinking about how much it hurt my feelings. But I know that I have told a lot of people about that incident and that I do verbalize at least a lot about how much, how, what conflict it is for me to be trying to [pause] please her and never succeeding. Like I, I've said a couple of times to different people that her love for me is qualified. And that's really the way I think of it, it's kind of, like, a yes, but. "Yes, I love you, but I'd love you more **if**." Or, "Of course, I love you because you're my daughter, but as a person I think you're disgusting." And that's really the way I feel. I don't feel that she loves **meeeee** [pause]. She loves a composite of the memories she chooses to remember, and the daughter she wishes I was [pause]. It really doesn't have anything to do with [pause] me. And it hurts me. It really hurts me to try. I avoid talking about it with her because I [pause] when I try to explain and I try to make her see me through my eyes, like when I try to justify myself or something, I say "Mom, do you think I would do this if I thought it was wrong?" You know, like she's sitting up there judging me. And saying, "You're a slut, you're a nymphomaniac. You're only doing this because you need a room to stay in or whatever." This was, this was where she started that I always went to bed with a guy for a reason. For a place to stay in the city, or I don't know what reasons she's come up with.

T: But that's a terrific insult.

P: It's very insulting and I, when I try to say to her, "Mom, I do it out of choice," I didn't say it that way, I said, "Mom, did it occur to you that I might want to? That I might like it, that I might enjoy sex?" Or, I always assume that sex is the issue. I don't know. Anyway, I remember saying to her once that I enjoyed it and she assumed that if I enjoyed it that that meant I was a nymphomaniac. And that's an insult, too. And it still doesn't leave me any conscious choice. It doesn't, it doesn't mean that I've thought about it, that I've made any decision, that I know what I'm doing at all, it's like I'm driven.

T: Yeah, well it may be that your mother has a reluctance to see you completely grown-up and independent of her.

P: Of course, she does. Sure she does, and [pause] I mean the idea of wanting me to come home for the summer just shows.

The hour continued with further clarification of the ambivalent attachment between Janice and her mother. She talked about her tendency to compete with a surviving brother in order to get attention from her mother. She enjoyed it when her mother asked her to come home, knew that her mother was hurt by her leaving, but knew too that she would not return. Now that she was out here, away from her mother, with nothing tangible to fight against, she felt a loss of direction. At home she could disagree with her parents and be more sure of who she was. But, paradoxically, another of her reasons for leaving home was that she tended to agree with her parents too much and didn't like herself for that. She wanted to get away from them and see where she stood on her own, although since leaving she has felt as if lost at sea.

This work led to discussion of a wish that occurred to her after the death and before the funeral; that the return home for the funeral would become a time of idealized, positive reattachment to her mother. Immediately upon her arrival, she was disappointed. Her parents were late, and not there when her plane arrived. She had hoped that when they met, her mother would reach out and they could embrace and comfort each other. Instead:

P: She didn't, she didn't, uh [pause] I didn't either [laughs]. When I think about it now, and I think maybe that's what I wanted, you know, like you

reach out and you loop each other's arms, and you look into each other's
eyes. And, then you know, something has passed between you. And nothing like that happened and I didn't initiate it and she didn't initiate it and
we probably both hoped the other would [pause].

T: You probably both experienced the other one as standing back.
P: That's—this is, that seems to be so funny about my memory there. I can
remember Gordon, I can remember Dad, but I can't remember—I can't
picture Mom. I mean I can't tell you what any of the other ones were
wearing, but I can at least kind of **see** them. And I can hardly see her [pause]
I don't remember hugging her or anything [long pause].

TWELFTH AND FINAL THERAPY HOUR

It is not surprising that, around the issue of termination, she rep-
licated aspects of the relationship with her mother in the relationship
with the therapist. The possibility of more extended therapy had been
discussed with her. She began the last session by stating that she had
decided not to go on into treatment [with another therapist; part of the
brief time-limited therapy agreement] but to go off alone and think over
her problems. It was clear that she wished to be independent and not
influenced too much by a therapist. Her idea was to spend one or two
days a week in an empty office, writing out details about the issues in
her life, consciously using her habitual style of generalization, intellectualization, and isolation.

The wish to get away from her parents came up again, even in
this last hour. The therapist had once more commented on her defensive
posture of standing aloof, as if she were watching herself have psychotherapy. Here is her response:

P: And watching me have psychotherapy?
T: Sure. That doesn't mean you haven't been getting it, and doing it, and
being involved in it. But at the same time you also have at times stood back
from it and looked at it. Isn't that so?
P: Um-hm [pause]. Especially at first. I mean I was watching you.
T: Um.
P: And your methods, what were you thinking, what were you going to do
and how would you react to this, that, and the other thing [pause]. I haven't
felt that way as much lately. I feel like I'm always to a certain extent watching
to have to control myself, for sure [pause]. I mean, you know, watching
how well I succeed. Like, a couple of times ago I was close to crying and I
stood back and I watched my lip tremble and my voice shake and . . . I
was congratulating myself on two different things at the same time; one on

actually crying and one I'm, you know, the **brave drama**, the trembling lip and all that [long pause while crying]. I wish that I could [pause] get away from my parent's definition of me [said very slowly and contemplatively]. I've, I've a couple of times in my life I've had this incredible feeling of freedom when someone has told me that I didn't have to think or feel or act in such and such a way.

T: Um.

P: Like I've had a glimmering the last couple of days. First of all that I can define myself, which is a kind of exciting idea. I don't think I really believe it but, it's hovering on my horizon. But that, you know maybe, **maybe** I am not the person my parents have always told me I am. Maybe I am, uh, other things. Like just the one I'm thinking of is maybe I'm a creative person. Maybe I **am** different. Maybe I cannot—maybe I don't **have** to act the way people are supposed to act.

T: Yeah.

P: Maybe, maybe I always will be a little oversensitive, a little confused, a little whatever, and maybe that'll be okay, and maybe I can use that. Or, you know, maybe I will become incredibly well-balanced and all that, in my own way, for myself. The trouble with wanting to be well-balanced is that it kind of seems like it's just stifling the definition as my parents' definition 'cause there is a definition of a together person and, and it's like trying to stuff myself into another mold sort of finding out what my own mold is.

As she talked about termination, she expressed a yearning for an adult relationship with a woman:

P: I feel like I'm continually searching for a woman friend, I've always had a best friend, or a couple of best friends. Maybe with some of them I talk about different things but there's always that feeling of rapport. "You know what I mean. You're on my side." And I haven't really had that here [pause]. And uh, with her I think of, well with Mary I don't feel tired or exhausted or anything when we're talking and we can talk for hours without realizing time's gone by [pause]. And it's so nice. And she's one of the reasons that I kind of, one of the things I put on the plus side of my taking therapy for awhile. "Well, I have a friend to talk to now."

T: Yeah.

Later she talked more directly about her wish to be taken care of. She recounted her shock several weeks back at being reminded that there were only a few sessions left, and described feeling as though she was engaged in a long phone call and would not have enough time. She also said, "I wish I could get sick, and be in the hospital or go crazy and be in a mental hospital or, or, you know, not have to be responsible."

She spoke of her current feeling about the death of her brother: "It's kind of funny, one of the things I feel most finished about is what I said I came in here for, which is about Sam's death. I mean all this time I've come to be much more accepting about my feelings about his death. I still dream about him, but I've been glad dreaming about him. I've been glad to be getting flashes of him. Because it hasn't been with that feeling of avoidance, instant rejection, and everything."

The difference between the relationship with the therapist, who fostered her independence, and the relationship with her mother, who tried to define her, is seen toward the end of this final therapy hour. She talked again of her early doubts about the therapist.

P: . . . What I've doubted was you.
T: Yeah?
P: Whether you could uh do it, whether you could . . . [pause] understand what I was saying [pause] and not take sides and uh [pause] make me work, kind of, make me go further than what I could do by myself. Be perceptive, you know, just do all the things that you're supposed to do and [pause]. And I wasn't at all sure what to do [pause]. It's like I could have, I would have known if you had been doing just a formula or, or your impersonation of a shrink or something like that or you had been maybe you are coming at me from a theory. But, um [pause] I don't feel I don't feel like you've tried to put a definition on me.

POSTTHERAPY EVALUATION INTERVIEW

Two months after the end of therapy the patient was reevaluated by the same clinician who had seen her initially and recommended the brief therapy. Her report validated the importance of the homesickness theme and the specific version triggered by the funeral.

E: As you look back, what was your experience of the therapy in terms of what you think happened during that time?
P: [Very long pause] In twenty-five words or less? Um [long pause] what happened, what happened? [long pause] I found out some things. I learned so, about therapy. As far as my brother, my brother's death, which was what brought me in, um, I think it helped. I, I think I also found out like right away that, that I, that wasn't really what I wanted to deal with. That I wanted to just deal with everything and . . .
E: So, you came in worried that you weren't dealing with the feelings around your brother's death. That sounds like that spread out in other things for you then.

P: Um, hm. An . . . and as long as I was in therapy I wanted to cure everything all at once. Um, he . . . Dr. Jones and I talked about some reasons about why I wa . . . hadn't reacted "**right**" to my brother's death like especially at home when I hadn't cried and I had felt like people were expecting me to cry, especially my mother, ta da. And those reasons made a lot of sense to me and, and the sense, the making sense has spread to other areas in looking at my relationship with my family. For instance, why I don't get homesick, why I came out here in the first place, why I don't want to go home. You know, all this stuff is that I just, um, I, is 'cause the same reason why I wouldn't cry. It's 'cause I didn't wanta play their game. I didn't wanta be sucked back in. I'm still trying to, to be apart and be myself. And, so I can't [pause] I couldn't really let go. And, that made sense to me. I liked that a lot better than any of the explanations that I had come up with, which was like you didn't care, your sense of reality is so warped that you don't believe it um [long pause] all those kind of things.

E: So, you let go of blaming yourself for not feeling the pain . . .

P: Right. I found a, the nicest excuse that I could accept. I don't know if it's true but, I think it is true because it applies to other things, I mean as soon as I, as soon as that kind of clicked, I felt better about my mother and I became aware of how oversensitive, how I overreact to a lot of the things that she does and says. So, yeah, I let go and my brother's death felt like a more natural thing.

She indicated that she was happier in her job and had applied for an advanced training program. She felt she had done something right and had made a step forward. She had more sense of where she was going, and was thinking carefully about her relationship with Phillip. They were still together, and she still had doubts about the wisdom of this arrangement.

She reported increased self-regard and self-control, as shown in this excerpt from the second posttherapy evaluation interview done 11 months after the termination of therapy. This interview was again, not with the therapist but with the evaluating clinician.

E: I'd like to get your kind of general impression first.

P: It's been over a year. Um, I feel a lot more in control of myself and of my life than I did then. I don't, I don't know if you remember or anything but I felt, you know, not just thrown by his death but jus, just powerless in general like everything kind of fell apart and I feel like I'm, um, I know what direction I'm going in, I have plans, and I'm more able to deal with daily crisis and stuff and, in fact, I'm, I'm dealing with a major crisis in a way that I'm, feeling pretty good about. That major crisis was that I'm leaving my, the guy that I've been living with.

She described how she was doing well at work and in her advanced training program. She had improved her relationship with her parents and had been successfully assertive in asking them to provide money for her education without attaching any strings to it. She had moved out, away from Phillip, although they remained friends: "I'm feeling so much better about myself that I don't need as much security, and I'm more able to face the things I don't like about the relationship." She was actively working in her mind on problematic patterns in her interpersonal relationships. "I demand a lot out of any relationship I'm in. This is one thing that bugs me. I feel like I'm a failure at relationships."

She talked about how she was going to go home soon to participate with her family in the scattering of Sam's ashes. She was able to talk directly about the worry that she might be embarrassed by crying too much or not crying enough. She cried briefly and appropriately during the session while talking about her brother and how she would spend a small sum of his money that was a last gift, and like a special memento from him. She also reported her competitiveness with relatives and others as to who had had "the most special" relationship with the dead brother. She resented the closeness between one of Sam's roommates and her mother, since the death. Here is a brief excerpt:

P: I might be able, um, share more, of my true feelings with my family if I come to terms with, uh, my feelings about Sam before then, because, the way I have been picturing [it] I have seen the kind of just going up there hopelessly and indecisively and pretending, trying to do the right thing for the sake of them, and knowing I wasn't gonna do it right. I'd either cry too much or, or be too withdrawn. I feel like my mother kind of accused me of being too withdrawn, when I was home for the funeral, and, and I remember feeling relieved and one time I really broke down and cried, because at last I had done the right thing, but if I can come to terms with my feelings, maybe I won't be so worried about doing the right thing.

These remarks one year later indicate her ability to remain in contact with themes initially warded off and then dealt with in therapy.

SUMMARY

A complex constellation of ideas and feelings has been called the homesickness theme. At the beginning of therapy this theme emerged, in a disavowed and disguised form. During the therapy, as shown by the transcripts presented in this chapter, there was progressive unfolding of the different sets of meaning within this constellation.

The work done on this theme involved joint effort within a therapeutic alliance. The interventions by the therapist and the information conveyed by both the form and content of his communications, affected the flow of meanings by altering the state of the patient, by stabilizing her realistic self-images, by altering the play of her internal controls, and by labeling important ideas.

This intervention process assisted her own natural process of working through a complex set of information, a process already in motion before treatment, and one that would continue after treatment.

References

Agras, S.: *Behavior therapy of stress response syndromes*. Talk given at symposium on stress: Psychotherapy of Stress Response Syndromes. University of California, San Francisco, June 1974.

Alexander, F., and French, T.: *Psychoanalytic therapy*. New York: Ronald Press, 1946.

American Psychiatric Association: *Diagnostic and statistical manual of mental disorders (DSM-III)*. Washington, D.C., 1980.

Arlow, J.: Unconscious fantasy and disturbances of conscious experience. *Psychoanalytic Quarterly 38*: 1 27, 1969.

Balint, M., Ornstein, P. H., and Balint, E.: *Focal psychotherapy*. London: Tavistock, 1972.

Bannister, D. (ed.): *Issues and approaches in personal construct theory*. London: Academic Press, 1985.

Bartlett, F. C.: *Remembering: A study in experimental and social psychology*. Cambridge, England: Cambridge University Press, 1932.

Basch, M. F.: Psychoanalysis and theory formation. In *Annual of psychoanalysis*. Institute for Psychoanalysis (ed.). New York: Quadrangle, 1973.

Beck, A. T.: *Cognitive therapy and emotional disorders*. New York: International Universities Press, 1976.

Beck, A. T., and Emery, G.: *Anxiety disorders and phobias: A cognitive perspective*. New York: Basic Books, 1985.

Benjamin, L. S.: Use of structural analysis of social behavior (SASB) and Markov chains to study dyadic interactions. *Journal of Abnormal Psychology 88*: 303–319, 1979.

Berne, E.: *Transactional analysis in psychotherapy*. New York: Grove Press, 1961.

Berne, E.: *Games people play*. New York: Grove Press, 1964.

Bibring, E.: The mechanism of depression. In *Affective disorders*. P. Greenacre (ed.). New York: International Universities Press, 1953.

Blacker, K. H.: Tracing a memory. *Journal of the American Psychoanalytic Association 23*: 51–68, 1975.

Blanck, G., and Blanck, R.: *Ego psychology*. New York: New York University Press, 1974.

Bower, G. H., Black, J. B., and Turner, T. J.: Scripts in memory for text. *Cognitive Psychology 11*: 117–120, 1979.

Bower, K. S., and Meichenbaum, D.: *The unconscious reconsidered*. New York: Wiley, 1984.

Bowlby, J.: *Attachment and loss. Vol. 1: Attachment*. London: Hogarth Press, 1969.

Bowlby, J.: *Attachment and loss. Vol. 2: Separation: Anxiety and anger*. New York: Basic Books, 1973.

Bowlby, J.: *Attachment and loss. Vol. 3: Loss: Sadness and Depression*. New York: Basic Books, 1980.

Boyer, L. B., and Giovacchini, P. L.: *Psychoanalytic treatment of schizophrenic and character-ological disorders*. New York: Aronson, 1967.

Breuer, J., and Freud, S. (1895): *Studies on hysteria. Standard Edition 2*. London: Hogarth Press, 1957, pp. 1–323.

Caplan, G.: *An approach to community mental health*. New York: Grune & Stratton, 1961.

Carlson, R., and Carlson, L.: Affect and psychological magnification: Derivations from Tomkins script theory. *Journal of Personality 52*: 36–45, 1984.

Caston, J.: Manual on how to diagnose the plan. In *Research on the psychoanalytic process I: A comparison of two theories about analytic neutrality* (Bulletin #3). J. Weiss, H. Sampson, and J. Caston (eds.). San Francisco: Mount Zion Hospital and Medical Center, December 1977.

Charcot, J. M.: *Lectures on diseases of the nervous system*. G. Sigerson (transl.). London: New Sydenham Society, 1877.

Derogatis, L., Lipman, R., and Covi, L.: The SCL-90: An outpatient rating scale. *Psychopharmacological Bulletin 9*: 13–18, 1973.

DeWitt, K., Kaltreider, N., Weiss, D., and Horowitz, M. J.: Judging change in psychotherapy: The reliability of clinical formulation. *Archives of General Psychiatry 40*: 1121–1128, 1982.

Eagle, M. N.: *Recent development in psychoanalysis: A critical evaluation*. New York: McGraw-Hill, 1984.

Edelson, M.: *Hypothesis and evidence in psychoanalysis*. Chicago: University of Chicago Press, 1984.

Ellenberger, H. F.: *Discovery of the unconscious*. New York: Basic Books, 1964.

Ellis, A.: *Reason and emotion in psychotherapy*. New York: Lyle Stuart Press, 1962.

Endler, N. A., and Magnusson, D.: Toward an interactional psychology of personality. *Psychological Bulletin 83*: 956–974, 1976.

Erdelyi, M.: *Psychoanalyses: Freud's cognitive psychology*. New York: Freeman, 1984.

Erikson, E.: *Childhood and society*. New York: Norton, 1950.

Erikson, E.: The dream specimen of psychoanalysis. *Journal of the American Psychoanalytic Association 2*: 5–55, 1954.

Erikson, E.: The problem of ego identity. *Journal of the American Psychoanalytic Association 4*: 56–121, 1956.

Fairbairn, W.: *An object relations theory of the personality*. New York: Basic Books, 1954.

Federn, P.: *Ego psychology and the psychoses*. New York: Basic Books, 1952.

Fenichel, O.: *Problems of psychoanalytic technique*. D. Brunswick (transl.). New York: Psychoanalytic Quarterly, Inc., 1941.

Ferenczi, S. (1926): *Further contributions to the theory and technique of psychoanalysis*. London: Hogarth Press, 1950.

Fiske, S. T., and Taylor, S. E.: *Social cognition*. Reading, MA: Addison-Wesley, 1984.

Frank, J. D.: Therapeutic components of psychotherapy. *Journal of Nervous and Mental Disease 159*: 325–342, 1974.

Freud, A.: *The ego and the mechanisms of defense*. London: Hogarth Press, 1936.

Freud, A.: Difficulties in the path of psychoanalysis: A confrontation of past with present viewpoints. In *Writings of A. Freud*. New York: International Universities Press, 1969.

Freud, A., Nagera, H., and Freud, W. E.: Metapsychological assessment of the adult person. The adult profile. In *Psychoanalytic study of the child*. R. S. Eissler *et al.* (eds.). New York: International Universities Press, 1965.

Freud, S. (1900): The interpretation of dreams. In *Standard Edition 4*. London: Hogarth Press, 1953a, pp. 1–678.

Freud, S. (1905): Three essays of the theory of sexuality. In *Standard Edition 7*. London: Hogarth Press, 1953b, pp. 125–244.

Freud, S. (1912): Totem and taboo. In *Standard Edition 13*. London: Hogarth Press, 1955a, pp. 1–164.

Freud, S. (1920): Beyond the pleasure principle. In *Standard Edition 18*. London: Hogarth Press, 1955b, pp. 7–66.

Freud, S. (1912): The dynamics of transference. In *Standard Edition 12*. London: Hogarth Press, 1958a, pp. 97–109.

Freud, S. (1914): Remembering, repeating and working through. In *Standard Edition 12*. London: Hogarth Press, 1958b, pp. 145–157.

Freud, S. (1909): Family romances. In *Standard Edition 9*. London: Hogarth Press, 1959a, pp. 235–244.

Freud, S. (1923): The ego and the id. In *Standard Edition 19*. London: Hogarth Press, 1961.

Freud, S. (1926): Inhibitions, symptoms and anxiety. In *Standard Edition 20*. London: Hogarth Press, 1959b, pp. 77–178.

Gaarter, K.: Control of states of consciousness: Attainment through external feedback augmenting control of psychophysiological variables. *Archives of General Psychiatry*. 25: 436–441, 1971.

Gedo, J., and Goldberg, A.: *Models of the mind*. Chicago: University of Chicago Press, 1973.

Gill, M. M.: *Analysis of transference Vol. 1. Theory and technique*. (Psychological Issues monograph no. 53). New York: International Universities Press, 1982a.

Gill, M. M.: *Analysis of transference Vol. 2*. New York: International Universities Press, 1982b.

Greenson, R.: *Technique and practice of psychoanalysis*. New York: Hallmark Press, 1967.

Greenspan, S. I., and Cullander, C.: A systematic metapsychological assessment of the personality. *Journal of the American Psychoanalytic Association* 21: 303–327, 1973.

Guntrip, H.: *Personality structure and human interaction*. New York: International Universities Press, 1961.

Haan, N.: *Coping and defending*. New York: Academic Press, 1977.

Hartley, D., Geller, J., and Behrends, R.: Manual for assessing developmental level of object representation. Langley Porter Institute, 1985 (unpublished).

Hartmann, H. (1950): Comments on psychoanalytic theory of the ego. In *Essays in ego psychology: Selected problems in psychoanalytic theory*. H. Hartmann (ed.). New York: International Universities Press, 1977.

Hartocollis, P.: *Borderline personality disorders*. New York: International Universities Press, 1977.

Horowitz, M. J.: Microanalysis of working through in psychotherapy. *American Journal of Psychiatry* 131: 1208–1212, 1974.

Horowitz, M. J.: *Stress response syndromes*. New York: Aronson, 1976. (2nd edition, 1986a.)

Horowitz, M. J.: Structure and the process of change. In *Hysterical personality*. M. J. Horowitz (ed.). New York: Aronson, 1977a.

Horowitz, M. J.: Cognitive and interactive aspects of splitting. *American Journal of Psychiatry* 134: 549–553, 1977b.

Horowitz, M. J.: *Image formation and cognition* (2nd ed.). New York: Appleton-Century-Crofts, 1978. (3rd ed., *Image formation and psychotherapy*. New Jersey: Aronson, 1983.)

Horowitz, M. J.: Psychological response to serious life events. In *Human stress and cognition*. D. Warburton and V. Hamilton (eds.). New York: Wiley, 1979.

Horowitz, M. J.: Self righteous rage and the attribution of blame. *Archives of General Psychiatry* 38: 1233–1238, 1981.

Horowitz, M. J., Levels of interpretation in dynamic psychotherapy. *Psychoanalytic Psychology* 3: 39–45, 1986b.

Horowitz, M. J.: *Introduction to psychodynamics.* New York: Basic Books, in press.

Horowitz, M. J., and Marmar, C.: The therapeutic alliance in difficult patients. *Psychiatry Update: American Psychiatric Association Annual Review Vol. IV,* 1985.

Horowitz, M. J., Marmar, C., Krupnick, J., Wilner, N., Kaltreider, N., and Wallerstein, R.: *Personality styles and brief psychotherapy.* New York: Basic Books, 1984.

Horowitz, M. J., Marmar, C., Weiss, D., DeWitt, K., and Rosenbaum, R.: Brief psychotherapy of bereavement reactions: The relationship of process to outcome. *Archives of General Psychiatry 41:* 438–448, 1984.

Horowitz, M. J., Marmar, C., Weiss, D., Kaltreider, N., and Wilner, N.: Comprehensive analysis of change after brief dynamic psychotherapy. *American Journal of Psychiatry 143:* 582–589, 1986.

Horowitz, M. J., Marmar, C., and Wilner, N.: Analysis of patient states and state transitions. *Journal of Nervous and Mental Disease 167:* 91–99, 1979.

Horowitz, M. J., Wilner, N., Marmar, C., and Krupnick, J.: Pathological grief and the activation of latent self images. *American Journal of Psychiatry 137:* 1157–1162, 1980.

Horowitz, M. J., and Zilberg, N.: Regressive alterations in the self concept. *American Journal of Psychiatry 140:* 284–289, 1983.

Horwitz, L.: *Clinical prediction in psychotherapy.* New York: Aronson, 1974.

Jacobson, E.: *The self and object world.* New York: International Universities Press, 1964.

Janet, P.: *The major symptoms of hysteria.* New York: Hafner, 1965.

Janis, I.: *Stress and frustration.* New York: Harcourt Brace Jovanovich, 1969.

Janis, I., and Mann, J.: *Decision making.* New York: Free Press, 1977.

Jung, C. G.: *The archetypes and the collective unconscious.* New York: Pantheon, 1959.

Kagan, R.: *The developing self.* Cambridge: Harvard University Press, 1982.

Kaltreider, N. B., DeWitt, K., Weiss, D., and Horowitz, M. J.: Patterns of individualized change scales. *Archives of General Psychiatry. 38* 1263–1269, 1981.

Karush, A.: Working through. *Psychoanalytic Quarterly 36:* 497–531. 1967.

Kelly, G. A.: *The psychology of personal constructs.* New York: Norton, 1955.

Kepecs, J. G.: Teaching psychotherapy by use of brief transcripts. *American Journal of Psychotherapy 31:* 383–393, 1977.

Kernberg, O.: *The borderline condition and pathological narcissism.* New York: Aronson, 1975.

Kernberg, O.: *Object relations theory and clinical psychoanalysis.* New York: Aronson, 1976.

Kernberg, O.: *Internal world and external reality: Object relations theory applied.* New York: Aronson, 1980.

Kiesler, D. J.: The 1982 interpersonal circle: A taxonomy for complimentarity in human transactions. *Psychological Review 90:* 185–214, 1983.

Klein, G. S.: Peremptory ideation: Structure and force in motivated ideas. In *Psychological Issues Vol. 5. Motives and thought: Psychoanalytic essays in honor of David Rapaport.* New York: International Universities Press, 1967, pp. 80–128.

Klein, G. S.: *Psychoanalytic theory.* New York: International Universities Press, 1976.

Klein, M.: *Contribution to psychoanalysis.* London: Hogarth Press, 1948.

Knapp, P. H.: Image, symbol and person. *Archives of General Psychiatry 21:* 392–406, 1969.

Knapp, P. H.: Segmentation and structure in psychoanalysis. *Journal of the American Psychoanalytic Association 22:* 14–36, 1974.

Kohlberg, L.: Stage and sequence: The cognitive developmental approach to socialization. In *Handbook of socialization theory and research.* D. A. Goslin (ed.). Chicago: Rand McNally, 1969.

Kohut, H.: Scientific activities of the American Psychoanalytic Association—An inquiry. *Journal of the American Psychoanalytic Association 18*: 462–487, 1970.

Kohut, H.: *Analysis of the self*. New York: International Universitites Press, 1971.

Kohut, H.: *The restoration of the self*. New York: International Universities Press, 1977.

Labov, W., and Fanshel, D.: *Therapeutic discourse*. New York: Academic Press, 1977.

Langer, S.: *Philosophy in a new key*. Cambridge: Harvard University Press, 1942.

Langs, R.: *The therapeutic interaction*. New York: Aronson, 1976.

Lazarus, R.: *The practice of multimodal therapy*. New York: McGraw-Hill, 1981.

Lazarus, R., and Folkman, S.: *Stress, appraisal and coping*. New York: Springer, 1984.

Loevinger, J.: *Ego development*. San Francisco: Jossey-Bass, 1976.

Loewald, H.: On the therapeutic action of psychoanalysis. *International Journal of Psycho-Analysis 24*: 16–33, 1960.

Luborsky, L.: Measuring pervasive psychic structure in psychotherapy: The core conflictual relationship. In *Communicative structures and psychic structures*. N. Freedman and S. Grand (eds.). New York: Plenum Press, 1977, pp. 367–396.

Luborsky, L.: *Principles of psychoanalytic psychotherapy: A manual for supportive-expressive treatment*. New York: Basic Books, 1984.

Mahler, M. S., Pine, F., and Bergman, A.: *Psychological birth of human infants*. New York: Basic Books, 1975.

Malan, D.: *A study of brief psychotherapy*. London: Tavistock Press, 1963.

Malan, D.: *Frontier of brief psychotherapy*. New York: Plenum Press, 1976a.

Malan, D.: *Toward the validation of dynamic psychotherapy*. New York: Plenum Press, 1976b.

Mann, J.: *Time-limited psychotherapy*. Cambridge: Harvard University Press, 1973.

Markus, H.: Self-schemata and processing information about the self. *Journal of Personality and Social Psychology 35*: 63–78, 1977.

Markus, H., and Smith, J.: The influence of self-schemata on the perception of others. In N. Cantor and J. F. Kihlstrom (eds.). *Personality, cognition and social interaction*. Hillsdale, NJ: Erlbaum, 1981.

Marmar, C., and Horowitz, M. J.: Phenomenological analysis of splitting. *Psychotherapy 23*: 21–29, 1986.

Marmar, C., Marziali, E., Horowitz, M., and Weiss, D.: The development of the therapeutic alliance rating system. In *The psychotherapeutic process: A research handbook*. L. Greenberg and W. Pinsoff (eds.). New York: Guilford Press, in press.

Marmar, C., Wilner, N., and Horowitz, M. J.: Recurrent patient states in psychotherapy: Segmentation and quantification. In *Process measures in psychotherapy research*. L. Rice and L. Greenberg (eds.). New York: Gulford Press, 1984, pp. 194–212.

Maslow, A. H.: *Toward a psychology of being*. Princeton: Van Nostrand, 1962.

Mayman, M.: Early memories and character structure. *Journal of Projective Techniques and Personality Assessment 32*: 303 316, 1968.

McLemore, C. W., and Benjamin, L. S.: What ever happened to interpersonal diagnosis. A psychosocial alternative to DSM III. *American Psychologist 34*: 17–34, 1979.

Meehl, P. E.: Why I do not attend case conferences. In *Psychodiagnosis: Selected papers*. Minneapolis: University of Minnesota Press, 1973.

Meichenbaum, D., and Gilmore, B.: The nature of unconscious processes: A cognitive behavioral perspective. In *The unconscious reconsidered*. K. S. Bower and D. Meichenbaum (eds.). New York: Wiley, 1984.

Menninger, K.: *Theory of psychoanalytic technique*. New York: Basic Books, 1958.

Mischel, W.: Cognition in self-imposed delay of gratification. In *Advances in social psychology*. L. Berkowitz (ed.). New York: Academic Press, 1973.

Modell, A. H.: A narcissistic defense against affects and the illusion of self-sufficiency. *International Journal of Psycho-Analysis 56*: 275–282, 1975.

Neimeyer, R.: Personal constructs in clinical practice. In *Advances in cognitive-behavioral research and therapy* (Vol. 4). P. C. Kendall, (ed.). New York: Academic Press, 1985.

Neimeyer, R.: *The development of personal construct psychology*. Lincoln: University of Nebraska Press, 1986.

Nisbett, R., and Ross, L.: *Human inference: Strategies and shortcomings of social judgement*. Englewood Cliffs, NJ: Prentice-Hall, 1980.

Norman, H., Blacker, J., Oremland, J., and Barrett, W.: The fate of the transference neuroses after termination of a satisfactory analysis. *Journal of the American Psychoanalytic Association 24*: 471–498, 1976.

Overall, J., and Gorham, D.: The brief psychiatric rating scale. *Psychological Reports 10*: 799, 1962.

Peterfreund, E.: Information systems and psychoanalysis: An evolutionary biological approach to psychoanalytic theory. *Psychological Issues 7*: Monograph 25/26, 1971.

Pfeffer, A. Z.: The meaning of the analyst after analysis. *Journal of the American Psychoanalytic Association 11*: 229–244, 1963.

Piaget, J. (1937): *The construction of reality in the child*. New York: Basic Books, 1954.

Pulver, S.: Can affects be unconscious? *International Journal of Psycho-Analysis 52*: 347–354, 1971.

Rangell, L.: A further attempt to resolve the problems of anxiety. *Journal of the American Psychiatric Association 16*: 371–404, 1968.

Rank, O.: *The trauma of birth*. New York: Harcourt Brace, 1929.

Rapaport, D.: *The organization and pathology of thought*. New York: Columbia University Press, 1951.

Rapaport, D.: Cognitive structures. In *Collected Papers of David Rapaport*. M. Gill (ed.). New York: Basic Books, 1967.

Rapaport, D., and Gill, M. M.: The points of view and assumptions of metapsychology. *International Journal of Psycho-Analysis 40*: 153–162, 1958.

Ryle, A.: *Frames and cages*. New York: International Universities Press, 1975.

Salzman, L.: *The obsessive personality*. New York: Science House, 1968.

Sampson, H., and Weiss, J.: *Research on the psychoanalytic process: An overview* (Bulletin #2). San Francisco: Mount Zion Hospital and Medical Center, March 1977.

Sampson, H., Weiss, J., and Gassner, S.: *Research on the psychoanalytic process II: A comparison of how previously warded-off contents emerge in psychoanalysis* (Bulletin #3). San Francisco: Mount Zion Hospital and Medical Center, December 1977.

Sampson, H., Weiss, J., and Mlodnosky, J.: Defense analysis and the emergence of warded-off mental contents: An empirical study. *Archives of General Psychiatry 26*: 524–532, 1972.

Schafer, R.: *Aspects of internalization*. New York: International Universities Press, 1968.

Schafer, R.: Internalization: Process of fantasy? *Psychoanalytic Study of the Child 27*: 411–436, 1972.

Schafer, R.: *A new language for psychoanalysis*. New Haven: Yale University Press, 1976.

Schank, R., and Abelson, R.: *Scripts, plans, goals, and understanding*. Hillsdale, NJ: Erlbaum, 1977.

Schilder, P.: *The image and appearance of the human body: Studies in the constructive energies of the psyche*. New York: International Unviersities Press, 1950.

Sifneos, P. E.: *Short-term psychotherapy and emotional crisis*. Cambridge: Harvard University Press, 1972.

Singer, J., and Salovey, P.: *Organized knowledge structures in personality: A review and research agenda*, in press.

Sperry, R. W.: Brain bisection and mechanisms of consciousness. In *Brain and conscious experience*. J. C. Eccles (ed.). New York: Springer-Verlag, 1966.

Spiegal, L. A.: The self, the sense of self and perception. *Psychoanalytic Study of the Child* 14: 81–109, 1959.

Spitz, R.: *The first year of life*. New York: International Unversities Press, 1965.

Stern, D. N.: *The interpersonal world of the infant*. New York: Basic Books, 1984.

Stevens, A.: *Archetypes: A natural history of the self*. New York: Morrow, 1982.

Strupp, H., Hadley, S., and Gomes-Schwartz, B.: *Psychotherapy for better or worse*. New York: Aronson, 1977.

Sullivan, H. S.: *The interpersonal theory of psychiatry*. M. L. Garvel and H. S. Perry (eds.) New York: Norton, 1953.

Taylor, S. E., and Crocker, J.: Schematic bases of social information processing. In *Social Cognition*. E. T. Higgens *et al.* (eds.). Hillsdale, NJ: Erlbaum, 1981.

Thickstun, J. T., and Rosenblatt, A. D.: *Modern psychoanalytic concepts in a general psychology*. New York: International Universities Press, 1977.

Tomkins, S.: Script theory: Differential magnification of affects. In *Nebraska Symposium on Motivation*. H. E. Howe (ed.). Lincoln: University of Nebraska Press, 1979.

Vaillant, G.: *Adaptation to life*. Boston: Little, Brown, 1977.

Vieth, I.: Four thousand years of hysteria. In *Hysterical personality* M. J. Horowitz (ed.). New York: Aronson, 1977.

Viney, T.: Self: The history of a concept. *Journal of the History of Behavioral Sciences* 5: 349–359, 1969.

Volkan, V. D.: *Primitive internalized object relations*. New York: International Universities Press, 1976.

Waelder, L.: The principle of multiple function. *Psychoanalytic Quarterly* 5: 45–62, 1930.

Wallerstein, R. S.: *Forty-two lives in treatment: A study of psychoanalysis and psychotherapy*. New York: Guilford, 1986.

Weiss, D., DeWitt, K., Kaltreider, N., and Horowitz, M. J.: A proposed method for measuring change beyond symptoms. *Archives of General Psychiatry* 42: 703–708, 1985.

Weiss, E.: *The structure and dynamics of the human mind*. New York: Grune and Stratton, 1960.

Weiss, J.: The integration of defenses. *International Journal of Psycho-Analysis* 48: 520–524, 1967.

Weiss, J.: Continuing research: The modification of defenses in psychoanalysis. *Journal of the American Psychoanalytic Association* 20: 177–198, 1972.

Weiss, J., Sampson, H., and Caston, J. (eds.): *Research on psychoanalytic process I: A comparison of two theories about analytic neutrality* (Bulletin 3). San Francisco: Mount Zion Hospital and Medical Center, December 1977.

Weiss, J., Sampson, H.: *Psychoanalytic process: Theory, clinical observation and empirical research*. New York: Guilford, 1986.

Wheelis, A.: *How people change*. New York: Harper & Row, 1973.

Wiggins, J. S.: A psychological taxonomy of trait-descriptive terms: The interpersonal domain. *Journal of Personality and Social Psychology* 37: 395–412, 1979.

Wiggins, J. S.: Circumplex models of interpersonal behavior in clinical psychology. In *Handbook of research methods in clinical psychology*. P. C. Kendall and J. N. Butcher (eds.). New York: Wiley, 1982.

Winnicott, D. W.: Transitional objects and transitional phenomena. *International Journal of Psycho-Analysis* 43: 89–97, 1953.

Index

Abreaction, 130, 131, 133
Acute self-disgust state, 22, 35–41, 49, 52,
    57–61, 63, 64, 92, 93, 187, 188
  complementary roles of, 63
  role relationships for, 103, 106, 107
Additional complaints, problems and, 22
Alliance, *see* Therapeutic alliance
Aloof state, 172–176
Analytic state, 179–181
Associations, 78, 79, 117, 118
Authentic working, 35, 37; *see also* Work-
    ing state
Awareness, 81, 118

Behavioral theory, 117
Bodily communication, 157, 202, 203
Borderline character configurations, 4, 25,
    30
Borderline personality, 193
Brief therapies, 119

Catharsis, 116, 117, 130, 131
Checking validity by microanalysis, 63,
    74–79, 109–113, 119, 131, 134–140
Cognitive-behavior therapy, 117
Cognitive maneuvers, interpretations of,
    202
Cognitive styles, 80, 81
Common state transitions, role relation-
    ship characteristics of, 58
Competitive state, 32, 37–41, 49, 60, 61,
    63, 92, 93, 95, 107, 135, 146, 147,
    187–189
Complex, 72
Conditioned associations, 117

Configurational analysis,
  applications of, during treatment, 195–
    205
  articulation with quantitative data, 192,
    193
  case vignettes, 170–176, 200
  in clinical investigation, 163, 191–193
  control groups and, 192
  defined, 4–8
  demographic variables, 192, 194
  evaluation interviews, 9
  events in, 8
  language and theory in, 3
  past therapy in, 13
  plan for, 1–18
  from process notes, 184
  psychological information in, 4, 200–203
  psychotherapy relationships in, 167–176
  reliability, 185, 186, 189–191, 194
  repetition in, 2
  research applications in, 185–195
  steps in, 4–7
  summary of, 4–8, 160, 161
  in teaching, 165–184
  tests for, 194
  typologies in, 193
Conflict, 74
Conflictual relationship schematization
    form, 65, 67, 69
  theme formulation, 66
Content analysis, 73, 185–195
Control modification
  information processing and, 115–141,
    179–181
  thought progression and, 116

Controls, 9, 71–88
    changes in, see Control modification
    failures, 74, 79
    ideational constellations, 74, 75, 159,
        160
    styles, 159
    therapist modifies, 124–141, 203, 204
Coping, 7, 78
Core conflictual relationship, Luborsky
    format, 66–68
Counteracting disavowal, 127–130
Crying-rage, 198, 199
Crying state, 32, 37, 39, 40, 42, 49, 60, 62,
    63, 92, 93, 147
    complementary roles, 63
    guilt and, 86
Cycles of states, modification, 91–95
    illustration, 92, 94

Decision making, 47, 77, 78, 116
Defenses, 156, 157, 203, 204
Defensive strategies, operations, 6, 64, 78,
    82, 200
Defensive style, shift in, 157, 159
Depression, ideas and emotions in, 79–88
Deprivation constellation, 178
Developmental level, 53
Diagnosis, role of, 25, 83
Dialogues, defined, 93
Dictionary of states, 27, 28, 42, 43
Directive techniques, 203, 204
Disavowal, counteracting of, 126–130
Dreams, 13, 158, 197
Drives, 72

Ego (self) development, 53
Ego psychology, 28–30, 49–56
Ego states, 29
Emotional states
    evocation of, 157
    microanalysis of, 83, 88
Emotions, theory of, 71–79, 115–141
Enduring attitudes, 74–77, 138
Events, in configurational analysis, 74–88
Externalization, 81, 83, 121, 130, 135, 176

Feelings, ideas and, 115, 141
Focus, 108–110, 216–219
Follow-up data, 17, 18, 173

Gedo–Goldberg system, 50–52
Generalization versus awareness, 81, 83
Giddy state, 198, 199
Grief work, 80
Group comparisons, 192, 193

Habitual styles, 6, 7, 79, 81, 83, 156
Hopkins Symptom Checklist, 22
Humiliation state, 172–176
Hurt and not working state, 31, 33, 39,
    40, 60, 62–64, 69, 84, 92–95, 135,
    146, 147, 187, 189, 223
    complementary image of, 63
    therapist and, 95, 122
Hurt but working state, 31, 32, 34, 36–41,
    49, 52, 56–59, 63, 92–95, 102, 103,
    106, 123, 134, 135, 138, 139, 147,
    187–190
    complementary image of, 63
    as major state, 198, 190
    therapist and, 95
Hysterical personality, 28, 193

Ideal goals, 151, 178
Ideal states, 35–37, 49, 63
Idealizing transference, 178, 182
Ideas, 71–88
    accessibility to consciousness, 156, 157
    conflicts and, 74
    conflictual or warded-off, 72, 73, 77, 79;
        see also Warded-off ideas
    constellations of, 78, 79, 85, 86, 153
    feelings and, 115–141
    illustration of, 79–88
    intrusive, 157
    microanalysis of, 83–88
    statement of, 78, 79
    status changes in, 156
Ideation, specific actions and, 75, 76
Ideational conflicts, models of, 73–74
Ideational constellations, 86
    change in, 156–161
    formulation of, 74–79
    microanalysis of, 83–88
    during therapy, 178
Ideational processing, 74
Identification, in psychotherapy, 170–176
Impaired by learning state, 56, 58, 59,
    103, 106

Information
  defined, 4
  identifying, 9
  pretherapy, change, and outcome in relation to, 7
Information processing, 3, 71–88
  applications of, 200–203
  change and, 118
  and change in controls, 179–181
  in configurational analysis, 1, 6
  and diagnosis, 83
  ideational and emotional conflicts in light of, 74–77
  illustration, 79–88
  microanalysis of, 83–88, 131–140
  modification of controls and, 114
  pattern descriptions and, 77, 78
  themes, 6, 7, 77, 78, 156
  in therapeutic process, 168–170
Information processing style, 176–183
  in awareness avoidance, 81, 83
  characteristic use of, 134, 135
Intention, 66
  ideas and feelings in relation to, 157
Interpersonal relationship, 5, 7, 12, 14
  pattern, 96–114
Interpretation, 118, 119, 191, 200
  levels, 120
  phases and their functions, 202
  reconstruction, abreaction and, 130, 131
  techniques, choice of, 203, 204
Intimate sharing state, 63, 64, 69
Intuition, 195, 196

Judgment, of developmental level, 51

Library of cases, 184
Life events, "serious" or "stressful," 75–77
Loevinger classifications, 53
Luborsky format, 66–68

Meaning, shifting of, 135
Microanalysis
  of information processing, 83–88, 131–140
  in listing of communications, 101
  plan for, 4–9
  of psychotherapy, 4–8
  of role relationships, 101, 109–114
  steps in, 4–7

Misalliance
  antithetical behavior and, 104
  negative transference and, 108
Models of the Mind (Gedo and Goldberg), 50
Modifying control, 115–141; see also Control modifications; Controls
  inhibition and, 125, 126
Monologues, 93
Multiple personalities, states in, 29
Multiple self-schemata, concept of, 45
Mutuality states, 172–176

Narcissistic personality disorder, 177
Negative transference, 198–214
Negative transference potentials, 104

Object concepts, 5, 44, 49–52
Object concepts versus self-concepts, 49–52
Object relations, diagnosis from, 49–52
Object schemata, see Object concepts
Obsessional character, 193
Oedipus complex, 46, 166
Optimal nontransference relationship, see Therapeutic alliance
Organizational level, self-, object schematization, 50–52
Outcome, 7
  description of, 143
  methods used in, 166, 167
  pluridetermined, 150
  role changes, 149–155
  state changes, 145–148
  style changes, 156–161
Overdetermination, 165

Past history, in configurational analysis, 11–13
Patient–therapist relationships, 93, 94, 171, 195–197; see also Transcript illustrations
  in configurational analysis, 3, 7
  development of, 96–114
  monologues and dialogues in, 93
  pretense in, 215, 216
  in psychotherapy, 97
Person schemata, 45, 52–55, 64, 68, 96
Personality, self-information and role relationship in, 17, 18

Plan diagnosis, 74
Play-acting state, 60
Pleasure, state altering and, 76, 77
Positive transference, 104–114
Posttherapy evaluation review, 260–262
Pretense, in patient–therapist relation-
    ships, 215, 216
Pretherapy period
    hurt and not working state and, 146
    self-disgust in, 146
Pretherapy states, changes in, 26–31, 145
Problem list, 5, 79
    defined, 21, 22
    format of, 21–25
    sample, 23, 166
Problems, 5
    additional complaints and, 22
    description of, 21–25
    diagnosis of, 25
    ideas and feelings in, 121
    illustrations of, 22–25
Process notes, 119, 184
Psychic environment, state, relationship,
    and information roles in, 4
Psychodynamic psychology, working state
    and, 198
Psychotherapy, see also Therapy
    analysis and microanalysis of, 4–8
    outcome in, 143, 151, 169, 170
    outlines for review of, 2–4
    sample case reviews, 166–170
    therapeutic relationship in, 97

Recurrent states, detailed observation
    about, 187
Regulatory maneuvers, see Controls
Relationship, 7
    defined, 4
    patient–therapist, see Patient–therapist
        relationships
    pretherapy change, and outcome in
        relation to, 7
Relationship conflicts, 6, 44, 65–68
Relationship models, 44–70, 149
Relationship patterns, 96–114
Relationship roles, defined, 45, 46
Reliability, 186–191
Repetition
    in configurational analysis, 2
    neurotic, 72
Repetition compulsion, 72

Research applications, 185–194
    in clinical investigations, 191–194
    reliability in, 186–191
Respondent idea, 74–77, 138
Reverie state, 177, 178, 180, 181
Righteous indignation state, 172–175
Role relationships, see also Relationship;
        Relationship models
    change in, 106
    in configurational analysis, 1, 5
    development of, 98–114
    illustration of, 56–63
    methods for describing, 52–64
    modeling of, 63
    models, 5, 7
    modification of, 149–155
    multiplicity of, 44–46
    self-concepts, 199, 200
    separate models of, 172–176
    transference, 98–114, 200–203
Role reversal, 100
Roles, see Role relationships

Self
    active and competent, 64
    as agent of action, 45
    definition, 43
Self-concept, 1, 5, 7, 45, 46, 48–52, 213,
        214; see also Self-images
    defective, 46, 167
    development of, 96–114
    methods for describing, 55–63
    models for, 199, 200
    role relationships and, 52–56
    stabilization of, 152
Self-development, milestones, 53
Self-disgust state, 57, 80, 81, 84, 85, 95,
        121–123, 135, 138, 146–148, 188, 189
Self-esteem, deflation of, 83
Self-images, 44–70; see also Self-concept
    changes in, 96
    cognitive style, 53
    complementarity of object images, 49–
        52
    complementary roles of, in relation to
        observed states, 63
    development of, 68, 96–114
    illustration of, 56–63
    modification of, 149–155
    multiple, 45
    personality and, 33

Self-images (*cont.*)
  pluridetermined outcome in, 150
  role relationship analysis in, 199, 200
  role relationship models and, 172–175
  working through ideas about, 175, 176
Self-representation, conflicts and, 65–68
Sequential dialogue
  laziness theme and, 127–130
  microanalysis of, 136, 137
Shame state, 61, 84, 85, 122, 123, 133
  role relationships form, 107
Shifting of meanings, 135
Signal anxiety, 72, 73
Silences, between therapist and patient,
  93, 94
Social alliance, 96, 98
State(s), 26–43
  acute despair, 62
  acute self-disgust, *see* Acute self-disgust
    state
  "as if," 49
  background of, 33
  change of, 4, 91–95
  closeness of observation, 36
  competitive, *see* Competitive state
  competitive-critical, 92, 93
  in configurational analysis, 1, 6
  crying, *see* Crying state
  cycle of, 38–41, 91
  defined, 4, 27, 28
  descriptive statements about, 189
  dictionary of aims, 27, 28
  dictionary of roles, 42, 43
  dictionary of states, 42, 43
  dissociative, 29
  frequency and quality of, 145–148, 193
  hurt and not working, *see* Hurt and not
    working state
  hurt but working, *see* Hurt but working
    state
  illustration of, 31–35
  intrusive crying, 166–169
  list of, 5, 32
  modulation, 30, 37, 42, 43
  multiplicity of, 27
  observation of, 36, 37
  and outcome, 7
  pretherapy, change, and outcome in
    relation to, 7
  quantification, 192, 193
  recurrent, 36

State(s) (*cont.*)
  relation of, to self-image, 49
  self-disgust, *see* Self-disgust state
  shame, 61, 84, 85, 122, 123, 133
  stability, 1
  "tra-la-la," *see* "Tra-la-la" state
  transactional analysis and, 29
  transition between, 28, 36–38, 56–63,
    91–95
  worthless or lost, 122
State analysis
  application of, during treatment, 197
  intrusive crying and, 167
  posttherapy, 145–148
  in psychotherapy, 171, 172
  quantitative method, 186–194
State definitions, 27–30
State descriptions, 26, 27, 30–32
  as elaborated by two judges, 187–189
  reliability of, 186–191
State identification, application of, during
    crisis treatment setting, 197–199
State transitions, 91–95, 103; *see also*
    States, transition between
  illustrations of, 92–94
  phases in, 94
  therapist intervention and, 94, 95
States of development, 68
Stress, 76, 80, 157
Stress event, 9, 108
Suggestion, 203, 204
Suicidal depression, 198, 199
Switching maneuvers, 81
  modification of, 126, 127, 158, 159
Symbolism, 181
Symptom, *see* Problems

Teaching, configurational analysis in, 165–
  184
Termination, 143
Tests, between patient and therapist, 93;
  see also Patient–therapist
  relationships
Thematic progression format, microanalysis, 83–88
Therapeutic alliance
  establishment of, 96, 98–114, 124, 169,
    200, 215, 221, 232, 237
  illustration of, 101–114
  microanalytic approach to, 100, 101,
    109–114

Therapeutic alliance (*cont.*)
  positive transference and, 104, 105
  role relationships in, 106, 109
Therapist, *see also* Patient–therapist
    relationships
  actions, 94, 95
  attributes, 92, 93
  in changes of state, 91–95
  effect of, on controls, 124–130
  intervention and change of state, 94, 95
  working models of, 195–197
Therapy, *see also* Psychotherapy
  changes in, 89, 90
  follow-up in, 143
  outcome of, 156–161
  thought, qualities of, 156–158
"Tra-la-la" state, 31, 32, 34–41, 49, 52, 56–
    60, 63, 64, 69, 84, 85, 92–95, 102–
    104, 106, 122, 125, 128, 133, 135,
    138, 139, 146, 147, 187–190, 221, 224
  complementary image of, 63
  as major state, 189, 190
  self-sufficiency and, 85
  therapist and, 95
Transactional analysis, 29, 30
Transcript illustrations, 215–262
  posttherapy evaluation interviews and,
    237–239, 260–262
Transference, 96, 181

Transference (*cont.*)
  erotic, 202
  interpretation, 97, 118, 200
  negative, 98–114
  positive, 104–114
  tests, 96, 99–101, 117
  variety of, 97
Transference gratification, 117, 204
Transmutative situation, 97, 118
Treatment, applications during, 195–205
Typologies, 193

Unconscious ideas, recording of, 116, 117
Unconscious plan, 74, 116
Unreliability in state descriptions, 185

Warded-off ideas, 72, 73, 77, 79, 117, 118,
    124, 158, 177–179, 201
  application of, 200–203
  working through, 181, 182
Warded-off state, 35, 36, 135
Wording, versus meaning, 110
Work experiences, in transcript illustra-
    tions, 226, 227
Working alliance, *see* Therapeutic alliance
Working models, utilization of, 195–197
Working state, 95, 123, 125, 128, 133, 138,
    146, 168, 169, 198, 199
Working through, 78, 115–141, 160, 175,
    176, 181, 182, 239–262